CBS—Quick Medical Examination Review Series

OPHTHALMOLOGY

SIXTEENTH EDITION

AF526874

Edited by :

DR. M.S. BHATIA (MD, Dip. WPA, MNAMS)
Professor & Head, Department of Psychiatry
University College of Medical Sciences
&
Guru Teg Bahadur Hospital,
Dilshad Garden, Delhi - 110095

Previously at :
Maulana Azad Medical College and Associated Hospitals, New Delhi
&
Lady Hardinge Medical College and Associated Hospitals, New Delhi

Contributing Editor :
DR. NIRMALJIT KAUR (MD)
Senior Specialist, Department of Microbiology
Dr. R.M.L. Hospital
New Delhi-110001

Previously at :
LHMC & Smt. S.K. Hospital, New Delhi

CBS

CBS Publishers & Distributors Pvt. Ltd.

NEW DELHI • BANGALORE • PUNE • CHENNAI • COCHIN (INDIA)

Dedicated to Readers Who Read, Understand & Reciprocate

ISBN : 978-81-239-2228-7

First Edition : 1992	Ninth Edition : 2000
Second Edition : 1993	Tenth Edition : 2001
Third Edition : 1994	Eleventh Edition : 2002
Fourth Edition : 1995	Twelfth Edition : 2003
Fifth Edition : 1996	Thirteenth Edition : 2004
Sixth Edition : 1997	Fourteenth Edition : 2005
Seventh Edition : 1998	Fifteenth Edition : 2010
Eighth Edition : 1999	Sixteenth Edition : 2012

Copyright © Authors & Publisher

All rights reserved. No part of this book may be reproduced or transmitted in any form or by any means, electronic or mechanical, including photocopying, recording, or any information storage and retrieval system without permission, in writing, from the publisher.

Published by Satish Kumar Jain and produced by V.K. Jain for
CBS Publishers & Distributors Pvt. Ltd.,
CBS Plaza, 4819/XI Prahlad Street, 24 Ansari Road, Daryaganj,
New Delhi - 110002, India. • Website: www.cbspd.com
e-mail: delhi@cbspd.com, cbspubs@airtelmail.in
Ph.: 23289259, 23266861, 23266867 • Fax: 011-23243014

Branches:

- ***Bengaluru:*** Seema House, 2975, 17th Cross, K.R. Road,
  Bansankari 2nd Stage, Bengaluru - 560070
  • Ph.: +91-80-26771678/79 • Fax: +91-80-26771680
  • E-mail: cbsbng@gmail.com, bangalore@cbspd.com
- ***Pune:*** Bhuruk Prestige, Sr. No. 52/12/2+1+3/2,
  Narhe, Haveli (Near Katraj-Dehu Road By-pass), Pune - 411051
  • Ph.: +91-20-64704058/59, 32342277 • E-mail: pune@cbspd.com
- ***Kochi:*** 36/14, Kalluvilakam, Lissie Hospital Road,
  Kochi - 682018, Kerala • Ph.: +91-484-4059061-65
  • Fax: +91-484-4059065 • E-mail: cochin@cbspd.com
- ***Chennai:*** 20, West Park Road, Shenoy Nagar, Chennai - 600030
  Ph.: +91-44-26260666, 26208620 • Fax: +91-44-42032115
  • E-mail: chennai@cbspd.com

Printed at : J.S. Offset Printers, Delhi

PREFACE

Life is a continuous learning process. Human beings are born to learn and gain knowledge. Education is a means to acquire knowledge and skills that an individual desires to practise. Examinations are the means to evaluate the knowledge. Though no method of evaluation is without flaw, the process of standardization has resulted in a multiple choice system of examination. This system satisfies the basic qualities of a measuring instrument viz., validity, reliability and objectivity.

Recently, a number of books have been published about these examinations but the **best book still remains that which covers the maximum number of questions, which had been asked in that particular examination,** because the chance of repetition of these questions from so-called **"Question Bank"** remains very high. Recently, it has been observed that many **"Question Banks"** have overlapped. So, it is best to do a book which is complete and covers the **"Question Banks"** of maximum number of examinations. This book is being forwarded in this direction.

This book is designed as a supplement to the standard textbooks. It includes the **Referenced - MCQ's** (of previous years papers) of various PG Medical Entrance and Services Examinations **speciality-wise and Chapter-wise** arranged. The students while preparing the text or just before the examination can quickly go through this book. This will help in detecting the areas of weakness in understanding the text and thus, will improve the skills with multiple choice system of examination. It is a favourite book for **"Paper-setters".**

The importance of doing MCQ's alongwith text has increased tremendously because, recently, it has become a tendency to frame MCQ's usually not covered by the standard textbooks followed at undergraduate level. **"Quick Medical Text Review Series"** can be a useful adjuant to this book.

Beware of the **Fraudulent Books** available in the market, which covers a part of copied '**Question Bank**' from this book, and also, based on '**Constructed**' rather than '**Original**' Question Book. It is suggested not to waste time on these books. Every MCQ matters a lot in a highly competitive exams.

I request the readers not to forget to send their opinions, as also suggestions and contributions if any, about all aspects of this book. It will be of invaluable help in enhancing the utility of the book in future.

All suggestions are welcome and will be duly acknowledged in future editions.

— Editors

A book of the Readers, for the Readers, by the Readers

NOTE

The MCQ's of multiple response type (i.e. with **more than one correct answer** have been omitted in this Edition. Kindly refer to separate books **(PGI MD Entrance Exam & DNB Entrance Exam.** Part-I) by the same author and Publishers.

ADVICE

Read carefully the suggestions in the beginning of this book.

Prepare text from books suggested in the beginning and go through **Referenced MCQ's** of this book. Don't waste time in inexperienced, **incomplete and fraudulent courses books for PG Medical Entrance Examinations.**

ABOUT THE BOOK

This book has been compiled with the main aim to help the students to **quickly revise the Chapter-wise up-to-date referenced question** asked in various entrance examinations (Years indicated in the brackets). **Quick Medical Examinations Review Series** contains Speciality-wise 45,000 MCQ's based on up-to-date papers from 1978 onwards.

The important examinations covered in this book (with code word in the bracket) are :

	Examinations	*Code used*
(A)	***All India level***	
1.	All India Postgraduate Entrance Examination	(AI)
2.	AIIMS MD Entrance Examination	(AIIMS)
3.	PGI MD Entrance Examination	(PGI)
4.	Combined Medical Services Examination by UPSC	(UPSC)
5.	Civil Services Entrance Examination, Part-I (Medicine)	(CS)
6.	Army Medical Corps Entrance Examination	(AMC)
7.	Diplomate of National Board Entrance Examination	(DNB)
8.	NIMHANS PG Entrance Examination	(NIMHANS)
9.	Sanjay Gandhi PG Institute Entrance Examination	(SGPGI)
10.	CIP Ranchi PG Entrance Examination	(CIP)
11.	Manipal Academy of Higher Education PG Entrance Examination	(Manipal/MAHE)
12.	Sree Chitra Tirunal Institute for Medical Science & Technology	(SCTIMST)
13.	Command Hospital, Bangalore	(CH)
14.	Bhabha Atomic Research Centre	(BARC)
15.	Institute of Aerospace Medicine	(IAM)
(B)	***State level***	
16.	Delhi MD Entrance Examination	(Delhi)
17.	Bihar MD Entrance Examination	(Bihar)
18.	JIPMER PG Entrance Examination	(JIPMER)
19.	CMC PG Entrance Examination	(CMC)
20.	Rohtak PG Entrance Examination	(Rohtak)
21.	MP State PG Entrance Examination	(MP)
22.	AP State MD Entrance Examination	(AP)
23.	TN State MD Entrance Examination	(TN)
24.	Karnataka Postgraduate Medical Entrance Examination	(Karnataka)
25.	Maharashtra PG Entrance Examination	(Maharashtra)
26.	Kerala State MD Entrance Examination	(Kerala)
27.	Rajasthan Postgraduate Entrance Examination	(Rajasthan)
28.	PG Entrance Examination, Varanasi	(BHU)
29.	Burdwan University	(BU)
30.	Combined Entrance Examination for PG Courses, U.P.	(UP)
31.	Punjab State PG Entrance Examination	(Punjab)
32.	Aligarh Muslim University PG Entrance Examination	(AMU)
33.	Nizam's Institute Entrance Examination, Hyderabad	(Nizam's)
34.	Postgraduate Admission Test, Orissa	(Orissa)
35.	Calcutta University Public Service Commission	(CUPSC)
36.	TN Public Service Commission	(TNPSC)
37.	Calcutta PG Entrance Examination	(Calcutta)
(C)	***Foreign***	
	PLAB, FCGP, GMC, FLEX, USMLE, MRCP, FRCS, MRCOG, etc.	

Sources of Errors (Ophthalmology)

Example 1 : **Rubeosis Iridis is seen in :** **AIIMS 1986, 88**

A. Diabetes mellitus
B. Eales disease
C. Retinoblastoma
D. Central retinal vein occlusion

Answer : All of the above are correct (Bhatia's Quick Medical Text Review. It is also seen in over 35 other causes). A wrongly framed Question. It should have contained **"most commonly seen in"** then answer would have been (A).

Example 2 : **Normal A : V ratio is :** **Delhi 1985**

A. 2 : 1
B. 1 : 2
C. 2 : 3
D. 3 : 2

Answer : Question was wrongly framed as it did not mention A : V ratio of *Fundus* and was included among Questions of General Medicine implying Atrio ventricular ratio.

Example 3 : **Cherry red macula is seen in :** **Rohtak 1986**

A. Retinal artery occlusion
B. Retinal venous occlusion
C. Multiple sclerosis
D. Taysach's disease

Answer : Both (A) & (D) are correct

Example 4 : **Earliest manifestation of Vitamin -A deficiency is :** **AIIMS 1985**

A. Night blindness
B. Xerosis
C. Bitot's spots
D. Keratomalacia

Answer : Earliest symptom (A) but earliest sign is (B)

Example 5 : **Diopteric power of human lens is :**

A. + 16 D
B. + 17 D
C. + 18 D
D. + 19D

Answer : Choice (B) in some books and choice (C) in some books.

Advice

Questions with inaccurate language (structuring) or wrong choices should better be left unattempted.

IMPORTANT OPHTHALMOLOGY TEXT FOR MCQ's

Examination	Examination of Eye, Ophthalmoscopy (direct & indirect), Retinoscopy Fundoscopy and Visual acquity (Snellen's test), Fluorescence angiography, Ultrasonography, ERG, VER
Optics	Types of Lenses (Convex, Concave, Cylindrical, Prism) and their uses, Contact lenses, IOL, Errors of refraction (myopia, hypermetropia, astigmatism, Presbyopia, Anisometropia), Reduced eye
Conjunctiva	Anatomy, Types of Conjunctivitis (membranous, ophthalmia neonatorum, angular, follicular, Viral), Trachoma, Phlyctenular and Vernal Conjunctivitis
Cornea and Sclera	Structure, Corneal ulcer, Leukoma, Hypopyon ulcer, Dendritic (interstitial keratitis), Keratoconus, Megalocornea, Episcleritis, Staphyloma
Chambers	Anterior and posterior, Mechanism of formation of aqueous
Uveal Tract	Pupil (Reflexes), Argyll-Robertson pupil (Classical & reverse type), Hutchinson's pupil, Causes of abnormalities (unilateral/bilateral, miosis/mydriasis), Iridocyclitis (D/D of red Eye), Vitreous
Lens	Anatomy, Cataract (Congenital, Senile, Diabetic, Complicated), Aphakia, Dislocation
Glaucoma	Definition and measurement of I.O. Pressure, Congenital glaucoma, Chronic Simple & Acute congestive glaucoma (Signs & treatment)
Retina	Anatomy, Eale's disease, Retinopathy (esp. in diabetes and hypertension), detachment, Retinoblastoma
Optic nerve	Anatomy, Amblyopia, Optic atrophy, Visual pathways (especially site of lesion and defect)
Strabismus	Squint, Nystagmus, Ocular nerve palsies
Eye Lids	Stye, Meibomian Cyst, Ectropion/Entropion, Ptosis, Dacryocystitis,
Miscellaneous	Proptosis, Vitamin-A deficiency, Injuries, (Symp. ophthalmia), Eye changes in systemic diseases, Operations (Lens extraction for glaucoma and ptosis). All named signs, tests and factual data

IMPORTANT TIPS OF OPHTHALMOLOGY

Read

* One must know about Normal Optic Data	Table in Bhatia's **Quick Medical Text Review**
* Lasers in Opthalmology	A.K. Khurana's **Ophthalmology**
* Everything about cataract	Parson's **Diseases of the Eye**
* Everything (especially signs and treatment) of Glaucoma	Parson's **Diseases of the Eye**
* About Special investigations of the Eye	Chatterjee's **Handbook of Ophthalmology,**
* Read about Contact Lenses	Bhatia's **Quick Medical Text Review**
* About Retinitis Pigmentosa	Parson's **Diseases of the Eye**
* Named Signs, Syndromes and Tests in Ophthalmology	Bhatia's **Quick Medical Text Review**
* About Ocular muscles (origin, action and nerve supply)	Chatterjee's **Handbook of Ophthalmology**
* About Drugs used in Ophthalmology	Table in Bhatia's **Quick Medical Text Review**
* About (Eighteen) causes of Angioid Streaks	Bhatia's **Quick Medical Text Review**
* About Intraocular lenses	Bhatia's **Quick Medical Text Review**
* About Ophthalmoscopy	Chatterjee's **Handbook of Ophthalmology**
* About operations for Cataract	Chatterjee's **Handbook of Ophthalmology**
* About twenty five causes of Cherry red spot in macula	Bhatia's **Quick Medical Text Review**
* About Retinopathies	Parson's **Diseases of the Eye**
* About visual pathways	Chatterjee's **Handbook of Ophthalmology**
* About Retinoblastoma	Bhatia's **Quick Medical Text Review**
* About Sympathetic Ophthalmia	Parson's **Diseases of the Eye**
* About Thirty seven causes of Rubeosis Iridis	Bhatia's **Quick Medical Text Review**
* Cryotherapy in Ophthalmology	A.K. Khurana's **Ophthalmology**
* Ocular embryogenesis	Parson's **Diseases of the Eye**
* Retinoscopy findings	Parson's **Diseases of the Eye**
* Types of Surgery for Myopia	Parson's **Diseases of the Eye**
* D/D of Red Eye	Parson's **Diseases of the Eye**
* Frequent causes of decreased Vision	Parson's **Diseases of the Eye**
* D/D of conditions producing visual loss with a normal fundus	Parson's **Diseases of the Eye**
* Ocular therapeutics	Parson's **Diseases of the Eye**
* Local anAesthesia in Ophthalmology	Parson's **Diseases of the Eye**
* Treatment of Aphakia	Parson's **Diseases of the Eye**
* Clinical Sign of Glaucoma	Parson's **Diseases of the Eye**
* D/D of optic nerve diseases	Parson's **Diseases of the Eye**
* One must know important points	Bhatia's **Quick Medical Text Review**

CONTENTS

1

IMPORTANT TEXT OF EXAMINATION

Types of pupillary reflex :

- * Cataracta nigra — Black
- * Cataracta brunescens — Brownish
- * Immature senile cataract — Greyish white
- * Mature senile cataract — Pearly white
- * Hypermature Morgagnian cataract — Milky white
- * Aphakia — Jet white
- * Calcium deposition — Chalky white
- * Glaucoma — Sea green

Purkinje Sanson images :

(Seen in darken room with candle light or pen torch)

- * 1st image — Anterior surface of cornea
- * 2nd image — Posterior surface of cornea
- * 3rd image — Anterior lens surface
- * 4th image — Posterior lens surface

Interpretation of Purkinje Sanson images :

- * 1st and 4th images — Clearly visible
- * 2nd and 4th images — Seen in bright light in darkrom
- * If 4th image is absent — Lens is opaque
- * If 4th image is present — Lens is clear
- * 3rd and 4th images — Aphakia (absence of lens)
- * 1st, 2nd and 3rd images move with the movement of light. — (Convex surfaces).

MCQ's OF EXAMINATION

What is important in Examination

Examination of Conjunctiva, Cornea, Lens, Retina, Ophthalmoscopy (direct & indirect), Retinoscopy and Visual acquity (Snellen's test)

1. **Tears are produced in the new born after : Delhi 1983; Bihar 1998**
   A. 1 week B. 2 weeks
   C. 3 weeks D. 4 weeks
2. **The acquity of distant central vision is tested at the following distance between the chart and the patient : Bihar 1998, 99**
   A. 10 meters B. 60 meters
   C. 6 meters D. 1 meters
3. **Fluorescein staining would be most useful in : DNB 1990**
   A. Bullous keratopathy
   B. Stromal dystrophies
   C. Corneal neovascularization
   D. Contact lens fitting
4. **Direct ophthalmoscopy is done for the examination of : Delhi 1998, 2000**
   A. Macula
   B. Field of vision
   C. Refracting media
   D. Determination of refraction
5. **In a patient with myopia and black floaters, cause is : PGI 1996**
   A. Glaucoma B. Lens dislocation
   C. Vitreous degeneration D. Retinopathy
6. **Aniscol's grid is used for : PGI 1996**
   A. Macular function
   B. Fundoscopy
   C. Measurement of IOP
   D. To detect retinal detachment
7. **In indirect ophthalmoscopy, following are seen except : AIIMS 1996, 99**
   A. Optic disc B. Periphery of retina
   C. Ora serrata D. Vitreous base
8. **In insulin dependent diabetes, sudden loss of vision is best investigated by : Delhi 1996, 98**
   A. Fundus immediately B. Refraction
   C. Perimetry D. Retinoscopy
9. **Specular microscopy is done for : Delhi 1996**
   A. Follicles B. Aqueous flare
   C. Vitreous opacities D. Corneal endothelium
10. **Megalocornea is seen in : AI 1996**
    A. Marchensani syndrome B. Turner's syndrome
    C. Wildervack's syndrome D. Horton's syndrome
11. **Unilateral optic neuritis most important finding : Jipmer 1997**
    A. Afferent pupillary degeneration
    B. Optic disc edema
    C. Optic congestion
    D. Opaque ocular media
12. **Photopsia occurs in : Karnataka 1996**
    A. Iritis B. Choroditis
    C. Cyclitis D. Scleritis
13. **Purely mydriatic (not cycloplegic) commercially available in our country : Orissa 1998**
    A. Atropine sulphate
    B. Cyclopentolate hydrochloride
    C. Tropicamide
    D. Phenylephrine hydrochloride
14. **A person with history of blunt trauma to the right eye 6 months back developed pain and circumcorneal congestion of the eye. The most important immediate investigation in this case is : AIIMS 1999**
    A. Intra-ocular tension
    B. Indirect ophthalmoscopy
    C. Posterior segment ultrasonography
    D. Angiography
15. **If retinoscopy (indirect) done at 1 m distance, lens used is - 1D. When performed at a distance of 50 cm, lens will be of : PGI 1999**
    A. +1D B. -2D
    C. -0.5D D. 1D
16. **Optic N. Axon emerges from : TN 1999**
    A. Ganglion cell layer B. Rods & cones
    C. Amacrine layer D. Nuclear layer

Ans. 1. A 2. C 3. D 4. A 5. C 6. A 7. D 8. A 9. D 10. A 11. A 12. B 13. D 14. A 15. C 16. A

17. ↑ DOT sign in fluorescent angiography is seen in : **UP 1999**
- A. Progressive macular oedema
- B. CSR
- C. Arteriovenous shunt
- D. Microaneurysms

18. Fundus examination should be done in maturity onset diabetes mellitus patient : **AIIMS 2000**
- A. At the time of diagnosis
- B. 10 yrs after diagnosis
- C. 15 yrs after diagnosis
- D. 5 yrs after diagnosis

19. Pachymeter is useful to : **Delhi 2001**
- A. Study corneal endothelium
- B. Study thickness of cornea
- C. Measure depth of anterior chamber
- D. Measure field of vision

Match the following (Ques. 20 to 24) :

20.	**Helmholtz**	A.	Astigmatism
21.	**Ruete**	B.	Direct ophthalmoscopy
22.	**Dallos**	C.	Contact lenses
23.	**Goldman**	D.	Indirect ophthalmoscopy
24.	**Thomas Young**	E.	Applantation tonometry & Gonioscopy

25. Hyperemia with blurred disc margins is seen in following except : **AP 1997**
- A. Hypermetropia
- B. Papilloedema
- C. Central Retinal Vein occlusion
- D. Retinitis Pigmentosa

26. Landolt's broken ring test is used for : **DNB 1989**
- A. Knowing the type of squint
- B. Recording visual acuity
- C. Charting the field of vision
- D. Testing the power of ocular muscles

27. For Superior orbital fissure, best view is : **AIIMS 1997**
- A. Plain AP view
- B. Caldwell
- C. Townes
- D. Basal view

28. Not true about Macular function test is : **AIIMS 1997**
- A. Two point discrimination
- B. Maddox rod
- C. Laser inferometry
- D. ERG

29. Cyclitic membrane is formed : **MAHE 1995**
- A. Anterior to the iris
- B. Anterior to the lens
- C. Behind the lens
- D. Behind the vitreous

30. The trichromatic theory of colour vision has been propounded by : **AIIMS 1983**
- A. Sloan
- B. Young Helmholtz
- C. Muller
- D. None of them

31. In retinoscopy using a plane mirror, when the mirror is tilted to the right the shadow in the pupil moves to the left in : **AIIMS 1983**
- A. Hypermetropia
- B. Myopia more than - 1 D
- C. Emmetropia
- D. Myopia less than - 1D

32. The electroretinogram may assist in the diagnosis of all of the following except : **AP 1988**
- A. Bilateral disease.
- B. Progression of retinal disease
- C. Clinically unsuspected disease in familial degenerations.
- D. Complications of glaucoma.
- E. Differentiation between peripheral and central retinal disease.

33. After retinal stimulation the visual impulse reaches occipital cortex after : **PGI 1981**
- A. 1 m sec.
- B. 24 m sec
- C. 124 m sec.
- D. 142 m sec.

34. Examination of the surface of cornea is done by : **Delhi 1998**
- A. Pachymeter
- B. Specular microscopy
- C. Gonioscope
- D. Corneotopography

35. The following are embryological remnants except : **AIIMS 1985, AMU 1986**
- A. Bergmeister's papilla
- B. Epicapsular stars
- C. Mittendorf's dot
- D. Posterior embryotoxon

36. Schwalbe's line is a continuation of : **PGI 1995**
- A. Descemet membrane
- B. Endothelium
- C. Stroma
- D. Epithelium

37. Orbital melanoma is best diagnosed by : **AMC 1994**
- A. Direct ophthalmoscopy
- B. Indirect ophthalmoscopy
- C. CT Scan
- D. ERG

38. Retinoscopy is used to study : **Rohtak 1996**
- A. Lesion of retina
- B. Lesion of macula
- C. Refractive errors
- D. Anterior chamber
- E. All of the above

39. To know the strength of intraocular lens used is : **Rohtak 1996**
- A. A scan
- B. B-Scan
- C. Retinoscopy
- D. Ophthalmoscopy

Ans.									
17. A	18. A	19. B	20. B	21. D	22. C	23. E	24. A	25. D	26. B
27. D	28. D	29. C	30. B	31. B	32. D	33. C	34. D	35. D	36. A
37. C	38. E	39. B							

40. **In Black floaters, investigation of choice is :** **PGI 1996**
A. Retinoscopy
B. Direct ophthalmoscopy
C. Indirect ophthalmoscopy
D. Slit lamp

41. **'A' wave in ERG corresponds to activity in :** **JIPMER 1993**
A. Rods B. Pigment epithelium
C. Inner retinal layer D. Nerve bundle layer

42. **Campimetry is used to measure :** **Delhi 1993**
A. Squint B. Angle of deviation
C. Pattern of retina D. Field charting

43. **All are true about ultrasonography of eye except :** **Rajasthan 1996**
A. Anterior surface of cornea, lens & retina can be seen
B. Intraocular tumour can be detected
C. Retrobulbar masses can be identified
D. Intraocular foreign body can not be localized

44. **Plasmoid aqueous may be produced by :** **DNB 1987**
A. Nitrogen mustard
B. Corneal application of eserine
C. Corneal application of histamine
D. Paracentesis
E. All of the above

45. **Direct ophthalmoscopy magnification of image in comparison to indirect type is ——— times.** **DNB 1990**
A. 2 B. 3
C. 5 D. 6

46. **Anomaloscope is used to detect :** **DNB 1990**
A. Squint B. Retinopathy
C. Congenital glaucoma D. Colour blindness

47. **Best diagnostic test for Best disease is :AIIMS 1983, 93**
A. Dark adaptation B. ERG
C. EOG D. Goniscopy

48. **Volume of an eye ball is approximately :** **AIIMS 1984, 89, 93**
A. 3 cc B. 5 cc
C. 7 cc D. 10 cc

49. **You are asked to examine the peripheral field of vision of a patient. On examination of the normal field, you expect to find decreased field of vision in which direction :** **AI 2002**
A. Upwards
B. Downwards
C. Looking towards right side (temporal)
D. Looking towards left side (Nasal)

50. **Which color would be best for foveal color testing :** **AI 2002**
A. Red and Green B. Blue and Green
C. Yellow and Green D. Red and Blue

51. **Tonography is important in :** **AI 2002**
A. Detecting the formation of aqueous humor
B. Detecting the drainage of aqueous humor
C. Gives continuous intraocular pressure tracings
D. Represents field changes

52. **For madox-rod test distance from patient should be (in meter) :** **Maharashtra 2000**
A. 0.5 B. 1
C. 2 D. 6

53. **20/20 vision means :** **CMC 2001**
A. 6/5 vision
B. American method
C. Criteria for blindness
D. Goal of India to become toper by 20/20
E. Programme for control of curable blindness

54. **Visual acuity in infants is tested with the help of :** **Maharashtra 2002**
A. Landolt's rings B. '4' dot test
C. Perimeter D. Slit lamp

55. **Photostress test is done to test :** **JIPMER 2003**
A. Macula B. Optic nerve
C. Refractive error D. Optic tract

56. **ICG angiography is primarily indicated in :** **AI 2009**
A. Minimal classical CNV
B. Occult CNV
C. Angioid streaks with CNV
D. Polypoidal choroidal vasculopathy

Ans. 40. D 41. A 42. D 43. D 44. E 45. B 46. D 47. C 48. C 49. A
50. A 51. B 52. D 53. B 54. A 55. A 56. B

EXPLANATIONS OF EXAMINATION

1. Ans.— A. 1 week
2. Ans.— C. 6 meters
3. Ans.— D. Contact lens fitting
4. Ans.— A. Macula
5. Ans.— C. Vitreous degeneration
6. Ans.— A. Macular function
7. Ans.— D. Vitreous base
8. Ans.— A. Fundus immediately
9. Ans.— D. Corneal endothelium
10. Ans.— A. Marchensani syndrome

    Megalo cornea is when diameter of cornea is more than 13 mm otherwise the eyeball is normal. In Microcornea, diameter of cornea is 12-13 mm. Refraction is hypermetropic. In megalocornea, diameter is about 16 mm. It is also called keratoglobus.
11. Ans.— A. Afferent pupillary degeneration
12. Ans.— B. Choroditis
13. Ans.— D. Phenylephrine hydrochloride
14. Ans.— A. Intra-ocular tension
15. Ans.— C. -0.5D
16. Ans.— A. Ganglion cell layer
17. Ans.— A. Progressive macular oedema
18. Ans.— A. At the time of diagnosis
19. Ans.— B. Study thickness of cornea
20. Ans.— B. Direct ophthalmoscopy
21. Ans.— D. Indirect ophthalmoscopy
22. Ans.— C. Contact lenses
23. Ans.— E. Applantation tonometry & Gonioscopy
24. Ans.— A. Astigmatism
25. Ans.— D. Retinitis Pigmentosa
26. Ans.— B. Recording visual acuity
27. Ans.— D. Basal view
28. Ans.— D. ERG
29. Ans.— C. Behind the lens

    Cyclitic membrane is formed in the anterior vitreous, behind lens due to organization of inflammatory exudate.
30. Ans.— B. Young Helmholtz
31. Ans.— B. Myopia more than - 1 D
32. Ans.— D. Complications of glaucoma
33. Ans.— C. 124 m sec.
34. Ans.— D. Corneotopography
35. Ans.— D. Posterior embryotoxon
36. Ans.— A. Descemet membrane
37. Ans.— C. CT Scan
38. Ans.— E. All of the above
39. Ans.— B. B-Scan

    In A-scan or time amplitude, radiosensitive A-block is used.
40. Ans.— D. Slit lamp
41. Ans.— A. Rods

    In ERG, A and B-wave are from photo receptors and the B-wave from Muller cells and C-wave originates in pigment epithelium. The ganglion cells do not contribute to ERG. The B-waves with a potential less 0.19 mV or more than 0.54 mV are considered abnormal. ERG is supernormal when the potential is above normal limits as seen in subtotal circulatory disturbance of retina; Subnormal when potential is less than 0.8mV. Negative, when a large A-wave is seen and positive 't' when an abnormal A-wave is followed by B-wave or absent B-wave, and Extinguished where in there is complete absence of response.

    A normal ERG record does not necessarily indicate normal retinal function. Advanced glaucoma, optic atrophy, Tay Sach's disease and macular disease may give normal response.
42. Ans.— D. Field charting

43. Ans.— D. Intraocular foreign body can not be localized.

44. Ans.— E. All of the above

Aqueous humour is a slightly alkaline clear, watery fluid with density higher than water. Volume in ant. chamber is 0.25 c.c. whereas that in the posterior chamber is about 0.06 c.c.

45. Ans.— B. 3

46. Ans.— D. Colour blindness

47. Ans.— C. EOG

48. Ans.— C. 7 cc

49. Ans.— A. Upwards

The normal visual field is upwards 60°, outwards more than 90°, downwards 70° and inwards 60°.

50. Ans.— A. Red and Green

In fovea contralis, only cones are present in neuroepithelial layer and other layers are almost completely absent.

51. Ans.— B. Detecting the drainage of aqueous humor.

Schiotz tonometer may be used.

52. Ans.— D. 6

53. Ans.— B. American method

54. Ans.— A. Landolt's rings

55. Ans.— A. Macula

56. Ans.— B. Occult CNV

* In a landmark article, Yannuzzi and associates demonstrated that ICG videoangiography was extremely useful in identifying well-demarcated localized areas of neovascularization in what had been classified as occult CNV by standard fluorescein angiography.

2

IMPORTANT TEXT OF OPTICS

PRISM

Definition—A prism is a medium, bounded by two plain refracting surfaces at an angle to each other.

This angle is called the ***angle of the prism*** and opposite the angle is the base of the prism.

Use of a prism—For treatment of heterophoria and for convergence insufficiency.

Spherical lens

Definition of a spherical lens—A spherical lens is a transparent medium bounded by spherical surfaces.

Usually thin lenses are used in ophthalmology.

There are mainly two types of spherical lenses—

Convex, converging or plus lens. It may be of three types :

(a) Double convex or biconvex

(b) Plano-convex

(c) Concavo-convex or convex meniscus

Use of a biconvex lens

A. For correction of hypermetropia

B. For correction of presbyopia

C. For correction of aphakia

Use of a biconcave lens—For correction of myopia.

Cylindrical lens

Cylindrical lenses are segments of a cylinder of glass cut parallel to its axis. Such a segment forms a convex cylindrical lens, whereas a similar segment from a mould in which the cylinder was cast, forms a concave cylindrical lens.

Use of a cylindrical lens—For correction of regular astigmatism

ERRORS OF REFRACTION, PRESBYOPIA AND ANISOMETROPIA

Errors of refraction

Emmetropia—It is the normal condition, when parallel rays of light from infinity come to a focus on the retina (fovea), when accommodation is at rest. Thus in emmetropia, there is no error of refraction.

Ametropia—It is a condition in which due to some refractive error, the parallel rays of light from infinity do not come to a focus on the retina (fovea), when accommodation is at rest.

There are three types of errors of refraction :

1. Myopia or short-sightedness
2. Hypermetropia or long-sightedness
3. Astigmatism

MCQ's OF OPTICS

What is important in Optics

Types of Lenses (Convex, Concave, Cylindrical, Prism) and their uses, Contact lenses, IOL, Errors of refraction (myopia, hypermetropia, astigmatism), Reduced eye

1. **In scotopic vision main role is played by: AP 1987, 95**
   A. Cones B. Rodes
   C. Both of the above D. Neither of the above
2. **Astigmatism is due to : PGI 1985; Rohtak 1986, 90**
   A. Axial ametropia B. Index ametropia
   C. Curvature ametropia D. Spherical abberation
3. **Cylindrical lenses are prescribed in: UPSC 1983**
   A. Presbyopia B. Astigmatism
   C. Myopia D. Squint
4. **The image in indirect ophthalmoscopy is: PGI 1983**
   A. Erect, virtual, magnified
   B. Erect, real, magnified
   C. Inverted, real, magnified
   D. Erect, virtual, normal
5. **The basic minimum illumination accepted for satisfactory vision includes: AP 1989**
   A. 15-20 foot candles
   B. 25-40 foot candles
   C. 40-50 foot candles
   D. More than 50 foot candles
6. **The law of refraction and reflection includes: AP 1988**
   A. Incident, reflected and refractive rays reside in the plane of incidence which is normal to the interphase.
   B. The angle of incidence equals the angle of reflection but has the opposite sign.
   C. Incident ray and refracted rays direction are related by the principle of Snell's law.
   D. All of the above.
7. **In an emmetropic eye, the magnification is X—— in the direct ophthalmoscope : DNB 1993**
   A. 5 B. 10
   C. 15 D. 25
8. **Direct ophthalmoscope projects : DNB 1989**
   A. Virtual, erect and magnified image
   B. Real, inverted and magnified image
   C. Real, erect and condensed image
   D. Virtual, inverted and condensed image
9. **Treatment of choice for high myopia is : JIPMER 1998**
   A. Contact lens B. Lensectomy
   C. YAG laser D. Spectacles
10. **Ophthalmoscope was invented by: AIIMS 1987**
    A. Donder (1940) B. Sherrington (1904)
    C. Goldman (1954) D. Babbage (1848)
11. **In hypermetropic eyes in children, the drug used tc dilate pupil is: AIIMS 1986, 87**
    A. Atropine B. Eserine
    C. Homatropine D. Any of the above
12. **A point that falls on the horopter is seen: AIIMS 1988, 95**
    A. Stereoscopically
    B. Double
    C. By corresponding retinal points
    D. With crossed diplopia
13. **Teichopsia is seen in: AIIMS 1986**
    A. Cataract B. Diabetes mellitus
    C. Multiple sclerosis D. Migraine
14. **Keratometry is done to: AIIMS 1986; PGI 1986, 87**
    A. Measure radius of curvature of cornea
    B. Measure thickness of cornea
    C. A.P. diameter of eye ball
    D. See lesions of optic disk
    E. Measure intraocular pressure
15. **Spherical abberation of the eye is decreased by : UP 1993**
    A. Cornea B. Lens
    C. Pupil D. Aquous humour

Ans.	1. B	2. C	3. B	4. C	5. A	6. D	7. C	8. A	9. B	10. D
	11. A	12. C	13. D	14. A	15. C					

16. 3 Purkinje Sanson Images are formed. Inverted image is seen on : AIIMS 1993
A. Anterior surface of cornea
B. Posterior surface of cornea
C. Anterior surface of lens
D. Posterior surface of lens

17. Pseudomyopia is seen in the cases of : Karnataka 1994
A. Acute congestive glaucoma
B. Diabetes mellitus
C. Chronic congestive glaucoma
D. Acute iridocyclitis

18. Vision centre is located in which lobe : Delhi 1994
A. Frontal B. Temporal
C. Parietal D. Occipital

19. Axial length of eyeball is —— mm. AI 1994
A. 16 B. 18
C. 24 D. 30

20. The following dimensions are correct except : AIIMS 1982, 85
A. The ora serrata is 6 mm from the limbus.
B. The mean axial length of the eye is 20 mm.
C. The cornea is approximately 0.5 mm thick centrally.
D. The equator is 16 mm from the limbus.
E. The radius of curvature of the anterior cornea is approximately 7.5 mm.

21. Visible spectrum extends from: JIPMER 1992
A. 100-300 mm B. 300-650 mm
C. 400-700 mm D. 720-920 mm

22. Facultative hypermetrotrophs manage to see because of: JIPMER 1992
A. Ciliary muscle contraction
B. Accommodation
C. Wrinkling of eye
D. Use of cycloplegica

23. Highest visual resolution is seen in : JIPMER 1992
A. Macula lutea B. Fovea centralis
C. Optic disk D. Ora serrata

24. Constantly changing refractive error is seen in: AIIMS 1992
A. Diabetic cataract B. Intumescent cataract
C. Morgagnian cataract D. Traumatic cataract

25. In myopia which one of the following is commonest: DNB 1991
A. Equatorial staphyloma
B. Posterior staphyloma
C. Ciliary staphyloma
D. Anterior staphyloma
E. Intercalary staphyloma

26. Which of the folowing has greater refractive power: AMU 1985; Kerala 1994
A. Anterior surface of cornea
B. Vitreous
C. Anterior surface of lens
D. Posterior surface of lens
E. Posterior surface of the cornea

27. Accommodation is maximum in: AMC 1990
A. Childhood B. Adulthood
C. Middle age D. Old age

28. A combination of flint and crown glass lenses produce: BHU 1985
A. An achromatic lens B. An applanatic lens
C. Both of the above D. None of the above

29. Ratio of magnification in distant direct ophthalmology to normal eye is : Delhi 1997
A. 2 times B. 5 times
C. 10 times D. 15 times

30. Photopic vision is due to: DNB 1989
A. Cones B. Rods
C. Both of the above D. Neither of the above

31. Protanopes cannot read : AIIMS 1985
A. Green B. Red
C. Blue D. Black

32. The size of the eye ball in myopia is : PGI 1983, 85; Delhi 1983
A. Bigger B. Smaller
C. Normal D. Can be of any size

33. Presbyopia is due to : AIIMS 1986
A. Loss of elasticity of lens capsule
B. Weakness of ciliary muscles
C. Weakness of suspensory ligament
D. All of the above

34. Diagnosis of Optic neuritis on Perimetry is by : Delhi 1988
A. Central Scotoma B. Peripheral Scotoma
C. Arcuate Scotoma D. Sickle shaped Scotoma

35. In emmotopic person, intraocular lens most commonly used has power of : Delhi 1995
A. + 18 D B. 19.5 D
C. 20.5 D D. 21.5 D

36. Keratoconus is best treated with —— lens. AIIMS 1983
A. Cylindrical B. Spherical
C. Convex D. Contact

37. In myopia, treatment of choice is : Rajasthan 1998
A. Nd laser B. YAG laser
C. Excimer surgery D. Argon laser

38. Near point of a 5-years old child is : Kerala 1998
A. 7 cms B. 10 cms
C. 15 cms D. 25 cms

Ans.										
	16. D	17. D	18. D	19. C	20. B	21. C	22. B	23. B	24. A	25. B
	26. A	27. A	28. C	29. B	30. A	31. B	32. A	33. D	34. A	35. A
	36. D	37. C	38. A							

39. **Shadow test is called :** **AMU 1987**
A. Gonioscopy
B. Retinoscopy
C. Direct ophthalmoscopy
D. Indirect ophthalmoscopy

40. **Kappa angle is the angle between the :** **AIIMS 1986**
A. Pupillary axis and optical axis
B. Visual axis and optical axis
C. Centre of eye-ball rotation and line of fixation
D. None of the above is correct

41. **Alpha angle axis and optical axis :** **AIIMS 1982**
A. Pupillary axis and optical axis
B. Visual axis and optical axis
C. Centre of eye ball rotation and line of fixation
D. None of the above

42. **Hemianopia is loss of :** **Delhi 1987**
A. One third of field
B. One half of field
C. One half of both nasal fields
D. One half of both temporal fields

43. **Anisometropia in children is corrected :** **Delhi 1986**
A. Partially B. Completely
C. Not at all D. By pleoptics

44. **If the size of the eyeball increases more than 24 min, it will cause :** **Delhi 1986**
A. Myopia B. Hypermetropia
C. Anisometropia D. None of the above

45. **Accommodation is controlled by :** **Delhi 1986**
A. Sphincter pupillae
B. Dilator pupillae
C. Ciliary muscle
D. Levator palpabral superioris

46. **3 year old with left eye seems larger than right, investigations to done are all except :** **PGI 1990**
A. Tonometry B. Gonioscopy
C. Ophthalmoscopy D. Perimetry
E. Retinoscopy

47. **Refractive index of tears is :** **DNB 1989**
A. 1. 13 B. 1.23
C. 1. 33 D. 1.37

48. **Concave lenses :** **MAHE 1996**
A. Are heavier than convex lenses
B. Make objects look larger
C. Are used to correct hypermetropia
D. Are represented by a negative sign

49. **Diopteric power of lens is :** **Delhi 1984, 85**
A. 16 B. 17
C. 18 D. 20

50. **An infant is born with :** **DNB 1985; Delhi 1985, 90**
A. Myopia B. Hypermetropia
C. Astigmatism D. Glaucoma

51. **If the size of the eyeball increases more than 24 mm, it will result in :** **Delhi 1998**
A. Myopia B. Astigmatism
C. Anisometropia D. Hypermetropia

52. **The radii of curvature of various refracting surfaces of the eye are as follows except :** **DNB 1990**
A. Anterior corneal surface + 5.5. mm
B. Anterior lens surface + 10.0 mm
C. Posterior corneal surface + 6.8 mm
D. Posterior lens surface +-6.0 mm
E. Anterior lens core : + 8.0 mm

53. **The accommodative convergence/accommodation ratio :** **AIIMS 1982, 85**
A. Is normally 3-5 : 1
B. Can be measured with the prism cover test
C. Is high in simulated divergence excess
D. Fixed ratio in each individual
E. Is low in hypermetropia

54. **The following are true of electroretinograms (ERGs) except :** **AIIMS 1986**
A. The ERG increases in size during dark adaptation.
B. The 'a' wave is negative.
C. The VER is reduced in amblyopia.
D. The 'b' wave of an ERG is altered out of proportion to the 'a' wave in retinitis pigmentosa.
E. The oscillatory potential is selectively abolished in patients with diabetic retinopathy.

55. **All visual reflexes are developed by :** **AI 1995**
A. 2 years B. 7 years
C. 10 years D. 12 years

56. **Snellen chart is used to test :** **Kerala 1994**
A. Vision B. Refraction
C. Presbyopia D. Amblyopia

57. **Aqueous flare is best demonstrated by :** **PGI 1993, 94**
A. Slit lamp examination B. Microscope
C. Torch light D. Direct ophthalmoscopy

58. **Lens used for indirect ophthalmoscopy is :** **PGI 1993, 94**
A. + 15 D B. + 22 D
C. + 30 D D. + 3 D

Ans.									
39. B	40. A	41. B	42. B	43. A	44. A	45. C	46. B	47. C	48. D
49. C	50. B	51. A	52. A	53. E	54. D	55. A	56. A	57. A	58. A

59. Astigmatism following cataract surgery can be prevented by all except : PGI 1993
A. Pre-operative keratometry
B. Small incision
C. Continuous suture
D. Sutureless surgery

60. A person doing retinoscopy in a patient with myopia sees with 1.5 D : PGI 1993, 94
A. Fast motion against B. Fast motion along
C. Slow motion against D. Slow motion along

61. Distant direct ophthalmoscopy is done at distance of : AIIMS 1994
A. 25 cm B. 50 cm
C. 20 cm D. 1 m

62. Most important factor determining convergence of light rays on retina : AIIMS 1995
A. Length of eyeball
B. Curvature of cornea
C. Diopter power of lens
D. Physical state of vitreous

63. Major amblyoscope is used for : Delhi 1995
A. Lateral Deviation of eye
B. Amblyopia
C. Ptosis
D. Exophthalmos

64. In retinoscopy at 1 m point of neutralization is achieved when far point of eye is : Delhi 1995
A. Behind the eye B. At fovea
C. 1 m in front of eye D. 6 m in front of eye

65. Lens used in presbyopia is : PGI 1996
A. Convex B. Concave
C. Bifocal D. Cylindrical

66. Mid point of eye ball is at —— mm. Rohtak 1995
A. 8 B. 10
C. 12 D. 14

67. Focussing on the retina is maximum done by : AI 1997
A. Cornea B. Lens
C. Aqueous D. Retina

68. Concommitant myopic (Divergent) Astigmatism is treated by : Rajasthan 1995
A. Orthoptic training
B. Instillation of atropine
C. Resection of lateral rectus
D. Resection of medial rectus

69. Lenticonus is seen in : AI 1996
A. Down's syndrome B. Alport's syndrome
C. Avellis syndrome D. Alstrom's syndrome

70. In Presbyopia, true are following except : WB 1996
A. Onset after age of 40
B. Loss of near sight
C. Recession of near point of distant vision
D. Common in hypermetropes than myopes

71. On retinoscopy at 1m distance there is no shadow, the eye is : AP 1996
A. Emmetropic B. 1 D myopic
C. 1 D hypermetropic D. Astigmatic

72. Following are refractive errors except : PGI 1997
A. Hypermetropia B. Myopia
C. Astigmatism D. Presbyopia

73. Ratio of magnification in distant direct ophthalmology to normal eye is : Delhi 1997
A. 2 times B. 5 times
C. 10 times D. 15 times

74. Treatment of choice for high myopia is : JIPMER 1998
A. Contact lens B. Lensectomy
C. YAG laser D. Spectacles

75. Astigmatism is : MAHE 1999
A. Spherical abberation
B. Curvature emmetropia
C. Axial emmetropia
D. Index emmetropia

76. A 35-years old man has near vision disturbance and distant vision 6/6. On retinoscopy at 1 m distance with +2 D sph. The diagnosis is : AIIMS 1999
A. Presbyopia
B. Accommodation paralysis
C. Ciliary spasm
D. Hypermetropia

77. The power of reduced eye is : TN 1999
A. 17 D B. 45 D
C. 59 D D. 66 D

78. Refractive condition of the eye at birth is : PGI 1999
A. Hypemetropia of 2 D
B. Myopia of 2D
C. Hypermetropia of 5 D
D. Myopia of 5 D

79. Which of the following units of measurement is employed to measure convergence. Kerala 2000
A. Dioptre B. Meter angle
C. Milimeter D. Prism dioptre
E. None of the above

Ans.									
59. A	60. A	61. A	62. B	63. A	64. C	65. C	66. B	67. A	68. D
69. B	70. A	71. B	72. D	73. B	74. B	75. B	76. D	77. C	78. A
79. B									

80. **A child was taken to the doctor by his mother, complaining that there is decrease in his school performance. His teacher says that he frequently squeezes his eyes and says that there is difficulty in seeing the blackboard. What is the most probable diagnosis : AIIMS 2000**
A. Myopia B. Hypermetropia
C. Presbyopia D. Astigmatism

81. **A 12 years old child with complaints of headache and decreased vision has a visual acuity of 6/36 in the right eye and 6/6 in the left eye. On Retinoscopy at 66 cms, the right eye showed correction of 1.5 D and left eye 5 D. The anterior chamber and fundus of the eye were normal. What may be the cause of decreased vision in the right eye : AI 2002**
A. Amblyopia B. Anisometropia
C. Optic neuritis D. Refractive error

82. **A patient, Om Prakash has hypermetropia and needs + 1.5 D glasses for distant vision. What would happen to his near vision when his glasses slip down his nose : AI 2002**
A. Gets distorted B. Remains unchanged
C. Becomes better D. Becomes worse

83. **Amblyopia should be corrected by : CUPGME 2002**
A. < 5 years of age B. 5-8 years
C. 8-12 years D. 10-15 years

84. **A patient with visual acquity of 6/60 but can see at 3/60 is having : DNB 2011**
A. Economical blindess
B. Social blindness
C. Manifest blindness
D. Absolute blindness

85. **Maximum refraction refractive index is of : DNB 2011**
A. Cornea B. Aquous
C. Lens D. Vitreous

86. **Air tear film is between : DNB 2011**
A. Len and aquous B. Cornea and aquous
C. Cornea and tear film D. Aquous and vitreous

Ans. 80. A 81. D 82. C 83. A 84. A 85. C 86. C

EXPLANATIONS OF OPTICS

1. Ans.— B. Rodes
2. Ans.— C. Curvature ametropia
3. Ans.— B. Astigmatism
4. Ans.— C. Inverted, real, magnified
5. Ans.— A. 15-20 foot candles
6. Ans.— D. All of the above
7. Ans.— C. 15
8. Ans.— A. Virtual, erect and magnified image
9. Ans.— B. Lensectomy
10. Ans.— D. Babbage (1848)
11. Ans.— A. Atropine
12. Ans.— C. By corresponding retinal points
13. Ans.— D. Migraine
14. Ans.— A. Measure radius of curvature of cornea
15. Ans.— C. Pupil
16. Ans.— D. Posterior surface of lens
17. Ans.— D. Acute iridocyclitis
18. Ans.— D. Occipital
19. Ans.— C. 24
20. Ans.— B. The mean axial length of the eye is 20 mm.
21. Ans.— C. 400-700 mm
22. Ans.— B. Accommodation
23. Ans.— B. Fovea centralis
24. Ans.— A. Diabetic cataract
25. Ans.— B. Posterior staphyloma
26. Ans.— A. Anterior surface of cornea
27. Ans.— A. Childhood
28. Ans.— C. Both of the above
29. Ans.— B. 5 times
30. Ans.— A. Cones
31. Ans.— B. Red
32. Ans.— A. Bigger
33. Ans.— D. All of the above
34. Ans.— A. Central Scotoma
35. Ans.— A. + 18 D
36. Ans.— D. Contact
37. Ans.— C. Excimer surgery
38. Ans.— A. 7 cms
39. Ans.— B. Retinoscopy
40. Ans.— A. Pupillary axis and optical axis
41. Ans.— B. Visual axis and optical axis
42. Ans.— B. One half of field
43. Ans.— A. Partially
44. Ans.— A. Myopia
45. Ans.— C. Ciliary muscle
46. Ans.— B. Gonioscopy
47. Ans.— C. 1. 33
48. Ans.— D. Are represented by a negative sign
49. Ans.— C. 18
50. Ans.— B. Hypermetropia
51. Ans.— A. Myopia
52. Ans.— A. Anterior corneal surface + 5.5. mm
53. Ans.— E. Is low in hypermetropia
54. Ans.— D. The 'b' wave of an ERG is altered out of proportion to the 'a' wave in retinitis pigmentosa.
55. Ans.— A. 2 years
56. Ans.— A. Vision
57. Ans.— A. Slit lamp examination
58. Ans.— A. + 15 D
59. Ans.— A. Pre operative keratometry
60. Ans.— A. Fast motion against
61. Ans.— A. 25 cm

62. Ans. — B. Curvature of cornea

63. Ans. — A. Lateral Deviation of eye

64. Ans. — C. 1 m in front of eye

65. Ans. — C. Bifocal

66. Ans. — B. 10

67. Ans. — A. Cornea

68. Ans. — D. Resection of medial rectus

69. Ans. — B. Alport's syndrome

70. Ans. — A. Onset after age of 40

71. Ans. — B. 1 D myopic

72. Ans. — D. Presbyopia

73. Ans. — B. 5 times

74. Ans. — B. Lensectomy

75. Ans. — B. Curvature emmetropia

76. Ans. — D. Hypermetropia

77. Ans. — C. 59D

78. Ans. — A. Hypemetropia of 2 D

79. Ans. — B. Meter angle

80. Ans. — A. Myopia

81. Ans. — D. Refractive error

82. Ans. — C. Becomes better

83. Ans. — A. < 5 years of age

84. Ans. — A. Economical blindess

Repeat Question

85. Ans. — C. Lens

Refractive index of cornea is 1.376 and those of aquous & vitreous humour is 1.336. Lens has refractive index of 1.406 (central layers) and 1.386 in less dense layers.

86. Ans. — C. Cornea and tear film

Repeat Question

3

IMPORTANT TEXT OF CONJUNCTIVA

ANATOMY AND DISEASES OF THE CONJUNCTIVA

Anatomy of the conjunctiva

Definition—The conjunctiva is a mucous membrane which covers the under surface of the lids and is reflected from the lids to cover the anterior part of the eyeball upto the margin of the cornea.

Different parts of the conjunctiva :

1. Palpebral conjunctiva—consisting of :
   (a) Marginal, (b) tarsal and (c) Orbital part
2. Conjunctiva of the fornix :
   It is the fold of the conjunctiva formed by the reflection of the mucous membrane from the lid to the eyeball.
3. Bulbar conjunctiva :
   It covers the anterior part of the eyeball upto the limbus
4. Conjunctiva of the limbus :
   It covers the limbus around the cornea.
5. Plica semilunaris :
   It is a crescentic fold of conjunctiva at the inner canthus, which is the rudiment of the nictitating membrane of lower vertebrates like frog.

CLASSIFICATION OF CONJUNCTIVITIS

A. *Infective conjunctivitis*—

1. *Conjunctivits due to bacterial infection* :

(a) Acute catarrhal or muco-purulent conjunctivitis—
   (i) Acute
   (ii) Sub-acute
   (iii) Chronic

(b) Membranous conjuctivitis

(c) Pseudo-membranous conjunctivitis

(d) Purulent conjunctivitis :
   (i) Gonorrhoeal conjunctivits
   (ii) Ophthalmia neonatorum

(e) Angular conjunctivitis

2. *Viral conjunctivitis* :

(a) Follicular conjunctivitis :
   (i) Acute
   (ii) Chronic

(b) Conjunctivitis in measles

(c) Conjunctivitis in varicella or chickenpox

(d) Conjuctivitis in herpes zoster ophthalmicus

(e) Conjunctivitis in variola

(f) Conjunctivitis in mumps

(g) Conjunctivitis in influenza

(h) Conjunctivitis in yellow-fever and dengue fever

(i) Conjunctivitis in vaccinia

3. *Conjunctivitis due to Bedsonia group of organism* :

(a) Swimming-bath conjunctivitis

(b) Trachoma

(c) Inclusion blennorrhoea of the new born.

4. *Conjunctivitis due to specific infections* :

(a) Tuberculous conjunctivitis

(b) Syphilitic conjunctivitis

(c) Tularensis conjunctivitis

(d) Conjunctivitis in leprosy

(e) Parinaud's conjunctivitis

B. ***Allergic conjunctivitis*** :

(a) Simple allergic conjunctivitis

(b) Phlyctenular conjunctivitis

(c) Vernal conjunctivitis of spring catarrh.

C. ***Conjunctivitis following injury***

D. ***Conjunctivitis associated with skin disease.***

DIFFERENTIAL DIAGNOSIS BETWEEN FOLLICULAR CONJUNCTIVITIS, VERNAL CONJUNCTIVITIS AND TRACHOMA

	Follicular Conjunctivitis	*Vernal Conjunctivitis*	*Trachoma Stages-I & II*
1. Seasonal variation	Nil	Present	Nil
2. Symptoms	Irritation with watering	Marked itching	Irritation with watering.
3. Follicles	Arranged in rows, never on plica.	No follicles	Irregular arrangement, may appear on the plica.
4. Papillae	None	Flat papillae cobble-stone	Fine papillae producing velvety appearance
5. Conjunctival discharge	Slight discharge —mucoid or than muco-purulent	Ropy discharge	Watery, mucoid discharge
6. Pannus	None	None	Always present
7. Corneal in-volvement	None	Sometimes an opacity, like arcus seniles	Corneal ulcers, followed by opacities.

THE RED EYE

	Conjunctivitis	*Anterior uveitis*	*Acute glaucoma*
Symptoms			
Pain	Minor-gritty or foreign	Present	Severe ocular pain and unilateral, frontal headache
Discharge	Present with stickness in morning	Absent	Absent
Vision	Unaffected	Blurred	Blurred-rainbow haloes around lights
Signs			
Hyperaemia	Superficial and diffuse most marked in fornices	Limbal	Diffuse and intense
Discharge	Mucoid, mucopurulent, or watery	Nil	Nil
Pre-auricular lymph node	Palpable	Impalpable	Impalpable
Cornea	Clear	Clear-but KP visible with slit lamp	Oedematous
Intraocular pressure	Normal	Occasionally elevated	High

MCQ's OF CONJUNCTIVA

What is important in Conjunctiva

Anatomy, Types of Conjunctivitis (membranous, ophthalmia neonatorum, angular, follicular), Trachoma, Phlyctenular and Vernal Conjunctivitis

1. **Trantas nodules are seen in : Delhi 1993**
A. Blepharoconjuctivitis
B. Vernal conjunctivitis
C. Phlyctenular conjunctivitis
D. Herpetic keratitis

2. **Organisms causing angular conjunctivitis is : Kerala 1986; Delhi 1992; PGI 2000**
A. Moraxella Axenfield bacillus
B. Pneumococci
C. Gonococci
D. Adenovirus

3. **Organisms causing ophthalmia neonatorum are except : Delhi 1992**
A. Neisseria Gonococci B. Staphylococci
C. Streptococci D. Neisseria meningitis

4. **Coloboma of the lid is commonest in the : Rohtak 1985**
A. Lateral half of the lower lid
B. Medial half of the lower lid
C. Medial half of the upper lid
D. Lateral half of the upper lid
E. Middle third of the lower lid

5. **Commonest cause of unilateral ptosis is : AMC 1986**
A. Orbital cellulitis B. Injury
C. Facial paralysis D. None of the above

6. **Typical coloboma of the iris appears in the : DNB 1986**
A. Upper part
B. Lower part
C. Nasal half of the iris
D. Temporal half of the iris

7. **All the following are true concerning squamous cell carcinoma of the conjunctiva except that : AIIMS 1981**
A. It is most commonly found at the limbus.
B. It has a strong tendency to infiltrate cornea either as a neoplastic process or as degenerative process i.e. pannus formation.
C. Tumors are highly radio sensitive.
D. 1/3 of these tumors will invade intraocular contents.

8. **Conjunctival xerosis may be seen in the following except : DNB 1990**
A. Pemphigus
B. Psoriasis
C. Steven Johnson disease
D. Sjogren's syndrome

9. **All of the following are true about Mooren's ulcer, except : AMU 1989**
A. Perforation is rare
B. Scar tissue replaces the damaged cornea
C. Undermined advancing border
D. Spreads centrally and centripetally

10. **Which of the following does not usually produce an inflammatory membrane : AIIMS 1986**
A. Steptococcus membrane
B. Diphtheria bacillus
C. Gonococcus
D. Haemophilus aegypticus (Koch-Weeks bacillus)

11. **The follicular conjunctivitis of adults associated with recent sexual exposure is : AMC 1984**
A. Moraxella lacunate
B. Inclusion blennorrhoea
C. Adeno virus and infection
D. New Castle disease virus conjunctivitis

12. **Chalazion is a chronic inflammatory granuloma of a : AMU 1985; TN 1993**
A. Meibomian gland B. Zies's gland
C. Sweat gland D. Wolfring's gland

Ans. 1. B 2. A 3. D 4. C 5. B 6. B 7. C 8. B 9. B 10. D
11. B 12. A

13. **Ophthalmia neonatorum is prevented by : TN 1989**

A. 1% Silver nitrate
B. Penicillin drops
C. Normal saline drops
D. Frequent eye washes

14. **Cornea is thinned in : Delhi 1989**

A. Keratoconus
B. Fuch's dystrophy
C. Bulbous lesion
D. All of the above

15. **Distichiasis is : DNB 1989**

A. An extra row of lashes
B. Central fusion of eye brow
C. Suturing of lashes
D. Absence of lashes

16. **Blindness in trachoma is due to : JIPMER 1997**

A. Loss of tear film
B. Cicatrical entropion
C. Pannus
D. Ptosis

17. **Subconjunctival haemorrhage may be seen in : AIIMS 1985, 86**

A. Mumps
B. Measles
C. Pertuseis
D. Rabies

18. **Incidence of trachoma is maximum in : AIIMS 1987**

A. Punjab
B. UP
C. Rajasthan
D. Orissa

19. **Epidemic keratoconjunctivitis transmitted by : PGI 1986, 90**

A. Hand shake
B. Eye-hand-eye
C. Droplet infection
D. Sneezing
E. Kissing

20. **Dendritic ulcer causing virus : PGI 1985, 90**

A. Herpes simplex
B. Herpes zoster
C. Cytomegalovirus
D. Adenovirus
E. Poxvirus

21. **Most common type of lid carcinoma is: AIIMS 1992**

A. Adeno carcinoma
B. Melanoma
C. Basal cell carcinoma
D. Squamous cell carcinoma

22. **Treatment of choice in angular conjunctivitis is: AIIMS 1992; PGI 1993**

A. Penicillin
B. Dexamethasone
C. Sulphacetamide
D. Zinc oxide

23. **Ptosis with lid lad is seen in: AIIMS 1992**

A. Congenital ptosis
B. Traumatic ptosis
C. Myogenic ptosis
D. Synkineses

24. **Herbert's pits are seen in: AIIMS 1992, 96; Delhi 1990, 99**

A. Trachoma
B. Herpetic conjunctivitis
C. Ophthalmia neonatorum
D. Spring catarrh

25. **Which of the following does not cause haemorrhagic conjunctivitis : AI 1995**

A. Adenovirus
B. Papilloma virus
C. Enterovirus 70
D. Coxsackie virus

26. **The H.P. inclusion bodies in trachoma are : Delhi 1987**

A. Intra-nuclear
B. Intra-cytoplasmic
C. Both
D. None of the above

27. **Symptoms of corneal ulcer are following except : AIIMS 1986**

A. Mucopurulent discharge
B. Pain in the eye
C. Redness of the eye
D. Watering

28. **Which of the following chemicals is not for tatooing of corneal opacity : AP 1988**

A. Gold chloride
B. Silver chloride
C. Platinum chloride
D. Hydrazine hydrate

29. **Follicles are not seen in which of the following : AIIMS 1983**

A. Spring cataract
B. Trachoma
C. Adenovirus conjuctivitis
D. Streptococcal

30. **All of the following result into loss of corneal sensations except : AIIMS 1983**

A. Acute congestive glaucoma
B. Absolute glaucoma
C. Dendritic ulcer
D. Mature senile cataract
E. Alcohol injection for trigeminal neuralgia

31. **Staphylococcus induced ocular complications are all except : PGI 1996**

A. Hordeolum
B. Phlyctena
C. Follicular conjunctivitis
D. Marginal infiltration of cornea

32. **Hordeolum externum is a suppurative inflammation of : AIIMS 1986**

A. Zeis' gland
B. Meibomian gland
C. Moll's gland
D. Gland of Krause
E. Gland Wolfring

Ans.									
13. A	14. A	15. A	16. C	17. C	18. A	19. B	20. A	21. C	22. D
23. C	24. A	25. B	26. B	27. A	28. B	29. A	30. D	31. C	32. A

33. **Intense itching is the most common symptom of : Kerala 1989**
A. Trachoma
B. Blephritis
C. Phlyctenular conjuctivitis
D. Spring catarrh

34. **Contraction and eversion of the conjuctiva of the eyelid is called : AIIMS 1982**
A. Coloboma B. Pterygium
C. Columella D. Ectropion

35. **In trachoma, mass treatment is given if a prevalence more than —— % severe or moderate trachoma in children below 10 years of age. Delhi 1996**
A. 1 B. 5
C. 10 D. 15

36. **The short posterior ciliary arteries are about —— in number. AMU 1988, 92**
A. 10 B. 20
C. 30 D. 40
E. 45

37. **Skin grafting of upper lid should be done ideally from : AIIMS 1982**
A. A split skin graft
B. A full thickness graft from behind the ear
C. Forehead rotation flap
D. Full thickness graft from forehand

38. **'Sago grain' follicles are characteristic of : PGI 1981, 86, 98**
A. Spring catarrh
B. Inclusion conjuctivitis
C. Phlyctenular conjuctivitis
D. Trachoma

39. **Which of the following is not a source of nutrients to cornea : AIIMS 1980**
A. Air
B. Aqueous humour
C. Perilimbal capillaries
D. Vitreous humour

40. **Treatment of phlyctenular conjunctivitis is : JIPMER 1997**
A. Systemic Anti-TB drugs
B. Systemic steroids
C. Topical acyclovir
D. Topical steroids

41. **The following are the features of conjunctival concretions except : TN 1989**
A. Calcification B. Palpebral location
C. Age related D. Corneal abbrasions

42. **As a complication of acute mucopurulent conjunctivitis, the corneal ulcers that develop are : AMU 1989**
A. Marginal B. Central
C. Anywhere on cornea D. No where

43. **Blood vessels in a trachomatous pannus lie : TN 1989**
A. Beneath the Descemet's membrane.
B. In the substantia propria.
C. Between Bowman's membrane & substantia propria.
D. Between Bowman's membrane & Epithelium.

44. **Dendritic ulcer is due to : PGI 1983**
A. Herpes simplex B. Fungal infection
C. Syphilis D. Phlycten

45. **"Orange skin" cornea results due to : AIIMS 1986**
A. Chalcosis B. Siderosis
C. Ammonia burn D. Mustard gas

46. **Refractive index of cornea is : Delhi 1989**
A. 1.30 B. 1.33
C. 1.37 D. 1.42
E. 1.50

47. **Increased visibility of corneal nerves is seen in : AP 1990**
A. Syphilis B. Leprosy
C. Onchocerciasis D. All of the above

48. **Following are seen in trachoma except : AIIMS 1997**
A. Epithelial keratitis
B. Stellate conjunctival scarring
C. Circumcorneal pannus
D. Conjunctival follicles

49. **Following are true about vernal conjunctivitis except : Delhi 1997**
A. Hypersensitivity reaction to exogenous allergens
B. Shield ulcer on cornea
C. Palpebral polygonal papilla with a flat top
D. Maxwell-Lyons sign positive

50. **Which of the following statements about herpes zoster ophthamicus is false: MAHE 1996**
A. It is caused by an RNA virus
B. Headache often precedes the rash
C. The cornea can be rendered anaesthetic
D. Glaucoma should be excluded

51. **In spring catarrh, seen is : Delhi 1988**
A. Phlyctena B. Epitheloid cells
C. Ropy secretion D. Pannus

Ans. 33. D 34. D 35. B 36. B 37. A 38. D 39. D 40. D 41. A 42. A
42. D 44. A 45. D 46. C 47. B 48. A 49. B 50. A 51. C

52. **Ophthalmia neonatorum occurs in : Delhi 1988**
A. 1-2 days B. 3-4 days
C. 4-7 days D. 7-14 days

53. **Not causing ophthalmia neonatorum : Delhi 1987**
A. Staphylococcus aureus
B. Adenovirus
C. TRIC
D. Gonococcus

54. **The dendritic corneal ulcer is typical of : Delhi 1985**
A. Varicella-Zoster infection
B. Herpes simplex infection
C. Pseudomonas infection
D. Aspergillus infection

55. **In vernal catarrh, the characteristic cells are : Delhi 1985, 87**
A. Macrophage
B. Eosinophils
C. Neutrophils
D. Epitheloid cells

56. **Trachomatous pannus is : Delhi 1987**
A. Vascular infiltration
B. Cellular infiltration
C. Epitheloid cells formation
D. Corneal opacity

57. **Ulcer serpens is most often caused by : AIIMS 1984**
A. Gonococcus B. TRIC
C. Pneumococcus D. Diphtheria

58. **Cobblestone appearance of conjunctiva is seen with : AIIMS 1986, 89, 94, 99**
A. Trachoma
B. Spring catarrh
C. Purulent conjunctivitis
D. Angular conjunctivitis

59. **Treament of choice of herpes conjunctivitis is : Delhi 1994**
A. Zidovidine B. Acyclovir
C. Ribovirin D. Ganciclovir

60. **Conjunctivitis is characterized by following except : Rajasthan 1998**
A. Pain B. Photophobia
C. Lacrimation D. Redness

61. **All are true about trachoma except : Kerala 1999**
A. Seen in unhygienic persons.
B. Follicle formation occurs in late stages.
C. The sequelae is decided by the complicating infection.
D. Pits are seen in the limbus in late cases.

62. **A new born baby of 2 days old with watery discharge in left eye with no edema, no pus or chemosis. Likely diagnosis is : AI 2000**
A. Chlamydial conjunctivitis
B. Gonococcal conjunctivitis
C. Chemical conjunctivitis
D. Ac. bacterial conjunctivitis

63. **In which of the following conditions in small ulcers the bleed are seen, on removing the yellow crusts on the lid margin : Kerala 2000**
A. Squamous blepharitis
B. Ulcerative blepharitis
C. Parasitic blepharitis
D. Hordeolum internum
E. All of the above

64. **In trachoma, all are seen, except : DNB 2001**
A. Ectropion B. Herbert's pits
C. Chalazion D. Corneal opacity

65. **Regarding spring catarrh, all of the following are true except : DNB 2001**
A. Cobblestone appearance of conjunctiva
B. Common in spring months
C. Limbus conjunctival thickening
D. Sodium cromoglycate is a form of therapy

66. **Conjunctivitis does not occur in : Kerala 2001**
A. CMV B. Adenovirus
C. Enterovirus D. Coxsackie virus

67. **Maxwell Lyon sign is seen in infection by : CMC 2001**
A. Spring catarrh
B. Dendritic ulcerative keratitis
C. Symphathetic ophthalmitis
D. Angular conjunctivitis

68. **Maximum density of goblet cells is seen in : AI 2004**
A. Superior conjunctiva
B. Inferior conjunctiva
C. Nasal conjunctiva
D. Temporal conjunctiva

69. **In which of the following conditions, severe itching of the eye with ropy discharge in a 10 years old boy with symptoms aggravating in summer season is most likely present : AI 2004**
A. Trachoma
B. Vernal keratoconjunctivitis
C. Acute conjunctivitis
D. Blepharitis

70. **Mass treatment with azithromycin is indicated if prevalence of trachoma follicles (TF) in 1-9 years populations is more than : AIIMS 2011**
A. 10% B. 8%
C. 6% D. 4%

Ans.									
52. A	53. B	54. B	55. B	56. A	57. C	58. B	59. B	60. A	61. B
62. B	63. B	64. A	65. C	66. A	67. A	68. C	69. B	70. A	

3.8 OPHTHALMOLOGY

71. **True about membranous conjunctivitis is : DNB 2011**
   A. Easy to peel
   B. If you peel, bleeding can occur
   C. Diphtheria causes false membrane
   D. Membrane can not be removed

72. **Phlyctenular conjunctivitis, not true is : DNB 2011**
   A. Hay fever most common cause
   B. Conjunctival edema
   C. Redness of eye
   D. Pain is rare

73. **Epidemic conjunctivitis is caused by : DNB 2011**
   A. Adenovirus
   B. Herpes virus
   C. EB virus
   D. Papilloma virus

74. **Child staying in dirty surroundings gets a pink nodule on conjunctiva with surrounding congestion, also has cervical and axillary lymphadenopathy. Diagnosis is : AI 2012**
   A. Phlyctenular conjunctivitis
   B. Allergic conjunctivitis
   C. Herpes keratitis
   D. Trachoma

Ans. 71. B 72. D 73. A 74. A

EXPLANATIONS OF CONJUNCTIVA

1. Ans.— B. Vernal conjunctivitis

   In bulbar conjunctivitis, presence of discrete whitish raised dots along the limbus are called Tranta's spots.

2. Ans.— A. Moraxella Axenfield bacillus
3. Ans.— D. Neisseria meningitis
4. Ans.— C. Medial half of the upper lid
5. Ans.— B. Injury
6. Ans.— B. Lower part

   Congenital coloboma (absence of tissue) of iris, ciliary body and choroid may be seen in association or independently. Typical coloboma is seen in the inferonasal quadrant and occurs due to defective closure of the embryonic tissue.

7. Ans.— C. Tumors are highly radio-sensitive
8. Ans.— B. Psoriasis
9. Ans.— B. Scar tissue replaces the damaged cornea
10. Ans.— D. Haemophilus aegypticus (Koch-Weeks bacillus)
11. Ans.— B. Inclusion blennorrhoea
12. Ans.— A. Meibomian gland
13. Ans.— A. 1% Silver nitrate

    Ophthalmia neonatorum is caused by chemicals (silver nitrate or antibiotics used for prophylaxis), gonococcal, staphylococcus, streptococcus, (neonatal inclusion conjunctivitis by) D to K chlamydial trachomatis and herpes simplex (II) ophthalmia neonatorum. The newborn closed eyelids should be thoroughly cleaned and dried. If infection is suspected a drop of silver nitrate solution 1% may be instilled into each eye (Crede's method). Chemical ophthalmia neonatorum is a self-limiting condition gonococcal (topical by bacitracin ointment 4 times or saline lavage, ceftriaxone or ciproflox systemically. For neonatal inclusion conjunctivitis 1% TC or 0.5% erythromycin and for herpes infection topical antiviral drugs are used.

14. Ans.— A. Keratoconus
15. Ans.— A. An extra row of lashes
16. Ans.— C. Pannus
17. Ans.— C. Pertuseis
18. Ans.— A. Punjab
19. Ans.— B. Eye-hand-eye
20. Ans.— A. Herpes simplex
21. Ans.— C. Basal cell carcinoma

    Rodent ulcer or basal cell carcinoma is the commonest malignant tumor of the lid. The commonest site is the lower lid, near the inner canthus. It originates either from the basal layer of epidermis or from the epithelium of the hair follicles and glands of skin.

22. Ans.— D. Zinc oxide

    Oxytetracycline (1%) eye ointment 2-3 times a day for 9-14 days will eradicate the infection. Zinc lotion during day and zinc oxide ointment at bed time inhibits the proteolytic ferment and thus helps in reducing the maceration.

23. Ans.— C. Myogenic ptosis
24. Ans.— A. Trachoma
25. Ans.— B. Papilloma virus
26. Ans.— B. Intra-cytoplasmic

    Chlamydia affects epithelial cells of cornea and the conjunctiva and produces inclusion bodies known as Hallber-steadter-Prowazek inclusion bodies. Leber cells, Arlt's line and Herbert pits are also seen.

27. Ans.— A. Mucopurulent discharge
28. Ans.— B. Silver chloride
29. Ans.— A. Spring cataract
30. Ans.— D. Mature senile cataract
31. Ans.— C. Follicular conjunctivitis

32. Ans. — A. Zeis' gland

Hordeolum externum or stye is a suppurative inflammation of one of Zeis's glands. Pain is considerable and hot compresses should be used in early stages. Incision is used when abscess find out. Antibiotic ointment may prevent recurrences.

33. Ans. — D. Spring catarrh

34. Ans. — D. Ectropion

35. Ans. — B. 5

36. Ans. — B. 20

Short posterior ciliary arteries have 10-20 branches. Long posterior ciliary arteries are two whereas anterior ciliary arteries are 7 in number.

37. Ans. — A. A split skin graft

38. Ans. — D. Trachoma

39. Ans. — D. Vitreous humour

40. Ans. — D. Topical steroids

41. Ans. — A. Calcification

42. Ans. — A. Marginal

43. Ans. — D. Between Bowman's membrane & Epithelium.

44. Ans. — A. Herpes simplex

45. Ans. — D. Mustard gas

46. Ans. — C. 1.37

47. Ans. — B. Leprosy

Dendritic ulcer is a typical lesion of recurrent epithelial keratitis due to herpes simplex virus.

48. Ans. — A. Epithelial keratitis

49. Ans. — B. Shield ulcer on cornea

50. Ans. — A. It is caused by an RNA virus

51. Ans. — C. Ropy secretion

52. Ans. — A. 1-2 days

Incubation period of various types of ophthalmia neonatorum is —chemical (4-6 hours), gonococcal (2-4 days), other bacterial (4-5 days), neonatal inclusion (5-14 days) and herpes simplex (5-7 days).

53. Ans. — B. Adenovirus

54. Ans. — B. Herpes simplex infection

55. Ans. — B. Eosinophils

56. Ans. — A. Vascular infiltration

57. Ans. — C. Pneumococcus

58. Ans. — B. Spring catarrh

59. Ans. — B. Acyclovir

Iodoxuridine (IDU) as 0.1% drops and 0.5% ointment or Acyclovir 3% ointment are used.

60. Ans. — A. Pain

61. Ans. — B. Follicle formation occurs in late stages.

62. Ans. — B. Gonococcal conjunctivitis

A watery discharge during the first week should be looked for gonococcal infection because tears are not secreted at this early age.

63. Ans. — B. Ulcerative blepharitis

64. Ans. — A. Ectropion

65. Ans. — C. Limbus conjunctival thickening

66. Ans. — A. CMV

67. Ans. — A. Spring catarrh

68. Ans. — C. Nasal conjunctiva

Goblet cells located within the epithelium and are most dense inferonasally.

Crypts of Henle are located along the upper third of the superior tarsal conjunctiva and along the lower-third of inferior tarsal conjunctiva.

Gland of Manz encircle the limbus.

69. Ans. — B. Vernal keratoconjunctivitis

Ropy discharge with symptoms aggravating in summer season are in favour of diagnosis vernalkerato conjunctivitis.

Vernal conjunctivitis (Spring catarrh):

- Caused by an immediate hypersensitivity reaction to some exogenous allergens.
- The disease has onset in summer months.
- Characterized by :
  - Intense itching, photophobia
  - White ropy discharge
  - Well-defined polygonal raised area of papillary hypertrophy on palpebral conjunctiva (cobblestone appearance).
  - Trantas spots (composed of degenerated eosinophilis) appear at limbus.
  - A stringy conjunctival discharge or a fibrinous pseudomembrane (Maxwell-Lyons sign) may some time be found.
- Treatment
- Sodium cromoglycate and steroid
- Iodoxamide tromethamine acts faster than sodium cromoglycate.

70. Ans. — A. 10%

If the baseline district prevalence of TF in 1-9-year-old children is 10% or greater, antibiotic treatment of all residents should be undertaken annually for 3 years. After these three treatments, a repeat district survey should be carried out.

71. Ans. — B. If you peel, bleeding can occur

Peeling cause bleeding.

72. Ans. — D. Pain is rare

Repeat Question

73. Ans. — A. Adenovirus

Group of adenoviruses cause.

74. Ans. — A. Phlyetenular conjunctivitis

It is a HS to bacterial antigens e.g. staph, T.B. etc. LN enlargement goes in favour of TB.

QUICK MEDICAL TEXT REVIEW SERIES

About this Series

- Comprehensive collection of **Important Text** subjectwise arranged
- This series include 20 books of Anatomy, Biochemistry, Physiology, Pharmacology, Microbiology, Forensic Medicine, Pathology, SPM, General Medicine, Psychiatry, Dermatology, Pediatrics, General Medicine, Orthopaedics, Anaesthesia, Ophthalmology, ENT, Gynaecology, Obstetrics and Radiology.
- Each book has been contributed by an *expert examiner of his field*
- This series is cost-effective supplement to the author's comprehensive book on MCQ's i.e. ***Quick Medical Examinations Review Series*** *(containing 40,000 MCQ's subjectwise)*
- **Important Topics** (for MCQ's and undergraduate examinations) in each subject has been listed in the beginning of each book to stress selective reading.
- There is no need to underline the books for MCQ's because important points to be remembered have been added at the beginning of each chapter.
- The books contains text from many standard textbooks of each subject
- Each book contains many important points and text usually **not covered by standard textbooks**
- Each series is presented with the hope and wish to invite fruitful interaction, comments, suggestions and contributions from its readers.
- Edited by : **Dr. M.S. Bhatia (MD; Dip. W.P.A., MNAMS)** - an experienced teacher and examiner who has worked in three leading Medical Colleges of Delhi (Maulana Azad Medical College, Lady Hardinge Medical College & University College of Medical Sciences) under Delhi University.
- Please send you suggestions and contributions to : **Dr. M.S. Bhatia,** D-1, Naraina Vihar, New Delhi - 110 028.

Keep your knowledge uptodate with this new series from:

CBS Publishers & Distributors Pvt. Ltd.

NEW DELHI • BANGALORE • PUNE • CHENNAI • COCHIN (INDIA)

4

IMPORTANT TEXT OF CORNEA & SCLERA

CORNEAL ULCER

Classification

A. Purulent ulcer or suppurative keratitis
   1. Ordinary pyogenic corneal ulcer.
   2. Hypopyon ulcer serpiginous ulcer of cornea.
   3. Mycotic ulcer.
   4. Marginal ulcer

B. Non-purulent ulcer
   1. Ulcer in association with trachoma
   2. Dendritic ulcer
   3. Lagophthalmic ulcer
   4. Ulcer due to vitamin-A deficiency
   5. Neurotrophic ulcer as produced by injection of alcohol in the Gasserian ganglion.

C. Allergic ulcer
   1. Phlyctenular ulcer

D. Degenerative ulcer
   1. Atheromatous ulcer occurring in old leucoma
   2. Mooren's ulcer

In general the ulcers occurring in the central area of the cornea are usually due to exogenous infection whether bacterial, viral or mycotic; those occurring in the periphery are often toxic or allergic in nature or due to endogenous infection.

Complications of corneal ulcer

1. Secondary glaucoma due to fibrinous exudation in the anterior chamber, which blocks the angle.
2. Perforation of the cornea with its sequelae.
3. Sloughing of the cornea with its sequelae.

Treatment

A. *Local*

1. Control of infection : Ideal method will be to detect the invading organism and its sensitivity to antibiotic cystalline penicillin 2,500 units with 0.5 gm of streptomycin sulphate dissolved in 1c.c of distilled water may be dropped every one hour, with a broad spectrum antibiotic ointment at bed time.

2. Rest to the eye :

(i) Atropine ointment 1 percent applied twice daily gives rest to the eye by paralysing the ciliary muscle. It also causes vasodilation and so bring more antibodies in the aqueous humour.

(ii) Dark glasses or shade to protect the eye from the irritating effect of strong light. But the eye must not be bandaged.

3. Relief of pain : Analgesics by mouth and hot compress.

Treatment of complications of corneal ulcer

a. For secondary glaucoma—paracentesis. Only hypopyon is not an indication for paracentesis.
b. For descemetocele when perforation is threatening—paracentesis and pad and bandage.
c. If perforation has occurred with iris prolapse—pad and bandage to prevent further iris prolapse
d. When the ulcer has sloughed off, with exposure of a good amount of iris, with or without the expulsion of the lens—pad and bandage with antibiotic ointment to be followed by enucleation later on when staphyloma has formed.

SCLERA

STAPHYLOMA

1. *Definition*—It is the ectasia of bulging of the wall of the eyeball along with uveal tissue.
2. *Types of staphyloma*

   a) Anterior staphyloma—as a result of sloughing of corneal ulcer.

   b) Ciliary staphyloma—due to bulging of the ciliary body due to thinning of the sclera, as a result of scleritis or injury to the sclera. This occurs in the area, extending upto 8 mm from the limbus. It is bluish in colour and irregular in appearance.

   c) Intercalary staphyloma—occurs at the limbus immediately in front of the ciliary body. Etiology is the same as for ciliary staphyloma.

   d) Equatorial staphyloma—occurs at the regions of sclera which are perforated by vortex veins and also a the equatorial region of sclera.

PSEUDOEPISCLERITIS (Lesions Resembling Episcleritis)

1. *Conjunctiva*
   A. Conjunctivitis
   B. Inflammed pinguecula
   C. Phlyctenular conjunctivitis
2. *Cornea*
   A. Punctate keratitis, such as that because of viral keratoconjunctivitis, Sjogren disease (secretoinhibitor syn drome), or psoriasis.
   B. Sclerosing keratitis because of scleritis.
   C. Rosacea keratitis associated with sector nebulae.
3. *Lids*
   A. In-growing lash
   B. Lash in punctum
4. *Metastatic carcinoma*
5. *Sclera,* such as scleritis with thinning
6. *Tumor,* such as malignant melanoma

BLUE SCLERA (Localized or Generalized Blue Coloration of Sclera Because of Thinness and Loss of Water Content Allowing Underlying Dark Choroid to be Seen)

1. Albright hereditary osteodystrophy (pseudohypoparathyroidism).
2. Bloch-Sulzberger syndrome (incontinentia pigmenti).
3. Brittle cornea syndrome (blue sclera syndrome)—recessive.

(Contd.....)

BLUE SCLERA (Localized or Generalized Blue Coloration of Sclera Because of Thinness and Loss of Water Content Allowing Underlying Dark Choroid to be Seen) (Contd...)

4. Corneal encroachment into sclera
5. Crouzon disease (craniofacial dysostosis)
6. de Lange syndrome (congenital muscular hypertrophy—cerebral syndrome)
7. Ehler-Danlos syndrome (fibrodysplasia elastica generalisata)
8. Folling syndrome (phenylketonuria)
9. Goltz syndrome (focal dermal hypoplasia syndrome)
10. Hallerman-Streiff syndrome (dyscephalia mandibulo-oculo-facial syndrome)
11. Hypophosphatasia (phosphoethanolaminuria)
12. Lowe syndrome (oculocerebrorenal syndrome)
13. Marfan syndrome (dystrophia mesodermalis congenita)
14. Osteogenesis imperfecta (van der Hoeve syndrome)
15. Paget syndrome (osteitis deformans)
16. Pierre-Robin syndrome (micrognathia-glossoptosis syndrome)
17. Pycnodysostosis
18. Relapsing polychondritis
19. Staphyloma
20. Turner's syndrome (gonadal dysgenesis)
21. Werner syndrome (progeria of adults)

DEEP ANTERIOR CHAMBER ANGLE

1. Normal variation
2. Aphakia
3. Myopia
4. Megalocornea or conical cornea including keratoconus
5. Congenital glaucoma
6. Posterior dislocation of the lens
7. Recession of anterior chamber angle

PHYSIOLOGIC MYDRIASIS (Dilated Pupil) (*Usually Greater than 5mm*)

A. Larger pupils in women than in men.
B. Larger pupils in myopes than in hypermetropes.
C. Larger pupils in blue irides than in brown irides.
D. Larger pupils in adolescents and middle-aged persons than in very young or old persons.
E. Voluntary dilatation (rare) by respiratory suspension and acceleration of heart beat.
F. Surprise, fear, pain, strong emotion, or vestibular stimulation.
G. General anaesthesia of stages-I, II, and IV.
H. Autosensory pupillary reflex—stimulation of middle ear.
I. Auditory pupillary reflex—tuning fork adjacent to ear.
J. Vestibular pupillary reflex — stimulation of labyrinth by heat, cold, or rotation.
K. Vagotonic pupillary reflex—stimulation on deep inspiration.

FIXED, DILATED PUPIL

1. *Midbrain damage*—vascular accidents, tumors, degenerative and infectious disease.
   A. Dorsal (Edinger-Westphal nucleus and its connections)—Rare involves both pupils, pupillary near vision reaction often retained, and often associated with supranuclear vertical gaze palsy.
   B. Ventral (fascicular part of third nerve)—Associated with other neurologic deficits, such as Nothangel syndrome, Benedict syndrome, Weber syndrome to spare the extraocular components of the third nerve.
2. *Damage to the third nerve* (from interpeduncular fossa to ciliary ganglion) :
   A. Basal aneurysms
   B. Supratentorial space—Occupying masses, causing displacement of the brain stem or transtentorial herniation of the uncus; stuporous or comatose.
3. *Damage to the ciliary ganglion or short ciliary nerves*—Results in Adie tonic pupil :
4. *Damage to the iris*
   A. Degenerative or inflammatory disease of the iris
   B. Posterior synechiae
   C. Acute rise of intraocular pressure (hypoxia or sphincter damage)
   D. Blunt injury to the globe with sphincter damage (traumatic iridoplegia)
   E. Pharmacologic blockade by atropinic substances.
5. *Total blindness,* including cortical blindness.

PHYSIOLOGIC MIOSIS (Small Pupil) (*Usually less than 2mm*)

A. Smaller pupil in men than in women.
B. Smaller pupil in hypermetropes than in myopes.
C. Smaller pupil in brown irides than in blue irides.
D. Smaller pupil in very young or old persons than in adolescents and middle-aged persons.
E. Sleep, fatigue, coma
F. Stage-III anaesthesia
G. Orbicularis reflex

Reader paratrigeminal syndrome—Ipsilateral miosis and pain—may by associated with third-nerve paralysis or corneal anaesthesia

A. Idiopathic B. Migraine
C. Meningioma D. Post-trauma
E. Extracranial aneurysm of internal carotid

ARGYLL ROBERTSON PUPIL—Small and irregular, reacts better to accommodation than to light

A. Syphilis (acquired lues)
B. Diabetes mellitus (Willis disease)
C. Chronic alcoholism
D. Different kinds of encephalitis
E. Multiple sclerosis (disseminated sclerosis)
F. Senile and degenerative diseases of the central nervous system
G. Midbrain tumors, such as pinealomas and craniopharyngioma
H. Friedreich ataxia
I. Malaria
J. Syringomyelia
K. Carbon disulfide poisoning
L. Herpes zoster, usually mydriasis
M. Pressure on third cranial nerve trunk by cerebral aneurysm
N. Trauma to skull or orbit
O. Abberrant regeneration of the third nerve

PERSISTENT PUPILLARY MEMBRANE

* = Most important

1. Fetal iritis
2. Hereditary
3. Physiologic
4. Use of oxygen therapy in premature nursery

DECENTERED PUPILLARY LIGHT REFLEX

1. Positive angle kappa—Pseudoexotropia
2. Negative angle kappa—-Pseudoesotropia
3. Eccentric fixation—Deep unilateral amblyopia
4. Ectopic macula—Macular displacement by retinal scarring or strands, such as retrolental fibroplasia
5. Ectopic pupil

PUPIL

The pupil is the circular aperture in the centre of the iris. The margin of the pupil rests on the anterior capsule of the lens. The pupillary aperture is controlled by the action of the dilator and the sphincter muscle. The normal size of the pupils is to **4 mm** in diameter.

Pupillary reflexes

1. ***Light reflex*** —
   a) Direct—The pupil contracts, as soon as light enters into the eye.
   b) Consensual—The pupil contracts, when light enters into the opposite eye.
   Afferent impulses from retina along the optic nerve and optic tract.
   Pretectal nucleus in the midbrain Edinger-Westphal nucleus of both sides.
   Efferent impulses via the 3rd nerve to the inferior the short root of the ciliary ganglion.
   Oblique muscle
   The ciliary ganglion short ciliary nerves
   The sphincter pupillae
2. ***Near reflex***—The pupil contracts on looking at a near object. It has two components :
   a) Convergence reflex, i.e., contraction of the pupil on convergence.
   b) Accommodation reflex, i.e., contraction of the pupil on accommodation.

MICROCORNEA (Cornea Having a Diameter of Less than 10mm)

1. Associated ocular findings :
   A. Aniridia and subluxated lenses
   B. Autosomal dominant cataract and myopia
   C. Autosomal dominant cataract, nystagmus and glaucoma
   D. Axenfeld syndrome (posterior embryotoxon)
   E. Colobomatous macrophthalmia
   F. Congenital glaucoma

G. Corectopia and macular hypoplasia
H. Hyperopia
I. Meckel syndrome
J. Non-ophthalmos
K. Narrow-angle glaucoma
L. Sclerocornea

2. Aberfeld syndrome (congenital blepharophimosis associated with generalized myopathy)
3. Autosomal recessive or dominant trait
4. Carpenter syndrome (acrocephalopolysyndactyly-II)
5. Chromosome 18 partial deletion (long-arm) syndrome
6. Ehlers-Danlos syndrome (fibrodysplasia elastica generalisata)
7. Gansslen syndrome
8. Hallermann-Streff syndrome (dyscephalia mandibulo-oculo-facialis)
9. Hemifacial microsomia syndrome
10. Hutchinson-Gilford syndrome (Progeria)
11. Laurence-Moon-Biedle syndrome (retinitis pigmentosa-polydactyly-adiposo-genital syndrome)
12. Lenz microphthalmia syndrome
13. Little syndrome (nail patella syndrome)
14. Locally associated with hyperopia, narrow-angle glaucoma, congenital glaucoma, or sclerocornea
15. Marchesani syndrome (mesodermal dysmorphodystrophy)
16. Marfan syndrome (dolichostenomelia-arachnodactyly-hyperchondroplasia-dystrophica mesodermalis congenita)
17. Meckel syndrome (dysencephalia splanchnocystic syndrome)
18. Meyer-Schnickerath-Weyers syndrome (oculodentiodigital dysplasia)
19. Rieger syndrome (hypodontia and iris dysgenesis)
20. Rubella syndrome
21. Sabin-Feldman syndrome
22. Schwartz syndrome (glaucoma associated with retinal detachment)
23. Trisomy 13-15 (D-trisomy)
24. Waardenberg syndrome (interoculoiridodermatoauditive dysplasia)

MEGALOCORNEA (Cornea Having a Horizontal Diameter of More than 14 mm)

1. Aarskog syndrome (facial digital genital syndrome)
2. Autosomal dominant or recessive trait
3. Congenital glaucoma (rare)
4. Marchesani syndrome (brachymorphy with spherophakia)
5. Marfan syndrome (dystrophia mesodermalis congenita)
6. Mucopolysaccharidoses I-S (Scheie syndrome)
7. Oculocerebrorenal syndrome (Lowe syndrome)
8. Oculodental syndrome (micrognathia-glossoptosis syndrome)
9. Osteogenesis imperfecta (van der Hoeve syndrome)
10. Pierre-Robin syndrome (micrognathia-glossoptosis syndrome)
11. Posterior embryotoxon
12. Rieger syndrome (hypodontia and iris syndrome)
13. Rubella syndrome (Gregg syndrome)
14. Sex-linked recessive trait
15. Sturge-Weber syndrome (meningocutaneous syndrome)

MCQ's OF CORNEA & SCLERA

What is important in Cornea & Sclera

Structure, Corneal ulcer, Leucoma, Hypopyon ulcer, Dendritic (interstitial keratitis), Keratoconus, Megalocornea, Episcleritis, Staphyloma

1. **A chronic iridocyclitis should be opened :** **BHU 1996, 99**
   A. Immediately
   B. Associated corneal ulcer
   C. If associated with glaucoma
   D. If it becomes acute
2. **The commonest organism responsible for corneal ulcer is :** **DNB 1990, 97**
   A. Staphylococci B. Pneumococci
   C. Pseudomonas D. Candida
3. **Band-shaped keratopathy is due to :** **AMU 1988**
   A. Calcerous degeneration B. Hyaline degeneration
   C. Fatty degeneration D. Elastotic degeneration
4. **Symptom differentiating scleritis from episcleritis is :** **Kerala 1989**
   A. Pain in eye B. Tenderness
   C. Discharge D. Lacrimation
   E. None of the above
5. **Ulcus serpens is caused by :** **TN 1996**
   A. Staphylococcus B. Streptococcus
   C. Pneumococcus D. H. influenza
6. **Ulcus serpens is caused in adults by :** **AIIMS 1980**
   A. Mycobacterium tuberculosis
   B. Streptococcus pneumoniae
   C. Corynebacterium diphtheriae
   D. Haemophilis influenzae
   E. All of the above
7. **Mechanism of Hypopyon ulcer formation :** **TN 1996**
   A. Exudation of toxins from iris & ciliary body.
   B. Direct pressure effect due to - IOT.
   C. Action of the inflammatory fluid on the corneal endothelium.
   D. None of the above.
8. **A hypopyon usually consists of :** **AIIMS 1982**
   A. Lymphocytes
   B. Polymorphonuclear leucocytes
   C. Polymorphs and causative organisms
   D. Infected pus
9. **Which of the following resembles cornea guttate :** **AIIMS 1986**
   A. Nodular corneal dystrophy of Groenouw
   B. Endothelial dystrophy of Fuchs
   C. Senile marginal degeneration
   D. Salzmann's corneal dystrophy
10. **The commonest cause of hypopyon is :** **Delhi 1985**
    A. Moraxella B. Gonococcus
    C. Pneumococcus D. Staphylococcus
    E. C. diphtheria
11. **Commonest cause of nodule at limbus is :** **Rajasthan 1994**
    A. Episcleritis B. Scleritis
    C. Phlyctena D. Pinguecula
12. **Most elastic and regenerable part of cornea is :** **Delhi 1988**
    A. Desmends B. Epithelium
    C. Endothelium D. Bowman's membrane
13. **Corneal transparency is due to all except :** **AIIMS 1986**
    A. Pump failure
    B. Normal IOT
    C. Hypercellular stroma
    D. Crystalloid arrangement of stroma
14. **Common cause of Exposure keratitis is :** **Rajasthan 1995**
    A. Tuberculosis B. Syphilis
    C. Leprosy D. AIDS

Ans.									
1. C	2. B	3. A	4. D	5. C	6. B	7. C	8. B	9. B	10. C
11. C	12. A	13. C	14. C						

15. Irrespective of the etiology of a corneal ulcer, the drug always indicated is : AIIMS 1985

A. Corticosteroid B. Atropine
C. Antibiotics D. Antifungal

16. Voisseus ring is seen in: AI 1993

A. Cornea B. Retina
C. Lens D. Anterior chamber

17. Ring scotoma is seen in: AI 1993

A. Retinitis pigmentosa B. Night blindness
C. Severe myopia D. Angle closure glaucoma

18. In case of central dense leucoma 5 mm Rx of choice is : AI 1993

A. Penetrating keratoplasty
B. Lamellar keratoplasty
C. Tattoing
D. Enucleation

19. Dense scar of cornea with incarcination of iris known as: AI 1993

A. Leukoma adherent B. Dense leukoma
C. Ciliary staphyloma D. Iris Bombe

20. Commonest earliest symptom of corneal ulcer is: Delhi 1993

A. Pain B. Watering
C. Gritty sensation D. Photophobia

21. Pseudohypopyon is seen in: Delhi 1993

A. Mycotic infection
B. Herpetic infection
C. Sympathetic ophthalmia
D. Trachoma

22. Which of the following organism can penetrate into the intact cornea: Delhi 1992

A. Pseudomonas B. Staphylococci
C. Diptheria D. Streptococci

23. Adhesion of iris margin anteriorly is known as: Delhi 1992

A. Intercalary staphyloma B. Anterior synychae
C. Posterior staphyloma D. Iris Bombe

24. Intercalary staphyloma is a type of : AIIMS 1983

A. Equatorial staphyloma B. Posterior staphyloma
C. Ciliary staphyloma D. Anterior staphyloma

25. Cornea is supplied by nerve fibres derived from: PGI 1984

A. Trochlear nerve B. Optic nerve
C. Trigeminal nerve D. Oculomotor nerve

26. Scleral ring: AIIMS 1982

A. Is the sclera round the cornea
B. Is ring shaped opacity in the cornea near limbus
C. Is pigmented ring in the sclera
D. Is a narrow white ring of the sclera round the optic disc
E. None of the above

27. Tuberculous keratitis shows: AMC 1984

A. Irregular panus
B. Heavy scar tissue
C. Response to topical corticosteroids
D. Invasion from the limus
E. All of the above

28. Which is not seen in corneal dystrophy : PGI 1996

A. Corneal opacification B. Corneal vascularization
C. White appearance D. None of the above

29. Features of megalocornea include all except: DNB 1991

A. Subluxation of lens is a frequent complication
B. Shallow anterior chamber
C. Cornea may be clear
D. Presence of embryotoxon at limbus

30. Corneal sensation is lost in -------- ulcer. AI 1996

A. Viral B. Fungal
C. Bacterial D. Hypopyon

31. Circumcorneal Congestion is not seen in : Delhi 1988

A. Herpetic keratitis B. Corneal ulcer
C. Phacomacular keratitis D. Catarrhal conjunctivitis

32. The following are involved in maintenance of corneal deturgescence except : PGI 1986

A. Hypertonicity of tear film caused by evaporation of water from the corneal surface.
B. Intraocular pressure.
C. Chloride transport across the epithelium.
D. Glycosaminoglycans.
E. Keratocytes

33. Interstitial keratitis is associated with all except : AIIMS 1983, 86

A. Measles B. Acquired syphilis
C. Tuberculosis D. Congenital syphilis
E. Leprosy

34. Keratoconus is associated with the following except : DNB 1991

A. Turner's syndrome
B. Leber's optic neuropathy
C. Aniridia
D. Thickened corneal nerves
E. Marfan's syndrome

35. Corneal deposits are seen in all except : Kerala 1994

A. Hunter's disease B. Hurler's disease
C. Eale's disease D. Coats retinopathy

Ans.										
	15. B	16. C	17. A	18. A	19. A	20. B	21. A	22. C	23. B	24. C
	25. C	26. D	27. E	28. D	29. B	30. A	31. D	32. E	33. A	34. B
	35. A									

36. **Not true about herpes keratitis :** **Delhi 1995**
A. Steroids acelerates recovery
B. Present in trigeminal ganglia
C. Recurrent
D. Usually unilateral

37. **Match List-I with List-II and select the correct answer using the codes given below the lists :** **UPSC 1995**

I. Dendritic ulcer	(i) Tubercular allergy
II. Leher's cell	(ii) Spring catarrh
III. Vernal conjunctivitis	(iii) Herpes simplex
IV. Phlyctenular conjunctivitis	(iv) Trachoma

Codes :

A. I (iii)	II (iv)	III (ii)	IV (i)
B. I (iii)	II (ii)	III (iv)	IV (i)
C. I (iv)	II (iii)	III (i)	IV (ii)
D. I (i)	II (iii)	III (iv)	IV (ii)

38. **Leucoria is seen in :** **Rajasthan 1989**
A. Glaucoma B. Cataract
C. Retinitis pigmentosa D. Acute dacryocystitis

39. **Most of the thickness of cornea is formed by :** **AMU 1987**
A. Epithelial layer B. Substantia propria
C. Descemet's membrane D. Endothelium

40. **Which type of corneal dystrophy is associated with acid mucopolysaccharidosis :** **PGI 1988, 95**
A. Granular B. Lattice
C. Macular D. Peripheral

41. **Sclera is about ------- mm thick at thickest portion.** **DNB 1990**
A. 0.2 B. 0.5
C. 1.0 D. 1.5

42. **Treatment of corneal abrasion with hypopyon is all except :** **AI 1994**
A. Systemic antibiotics B. Cautery
C. Atropine D. Corneal graft

43. **Satellite lesions are seen in Keratitis due to:** **AIIMS 1992**
A. HSV B. Herpes zoster
C. Aspergillus D. Pneumococcus

44. **Fasicular ulcer is present in:** **JIPMER 1993**
A. Mooren's ulcer B. Neuroparalytic keratitis
C. Herpes zoster D. Marginal ulcer

45. **Bullous keratopathy involves:** **AI 1993**
A. Descemet's membrane B. Epithelium
C. Endothelium D. Bowmen's membrane

46. **Iris Pearl is seen in :** **WB 1998**
A. Sarcoidosis B. TB
C. Leprosy D. Ankylosing spondylysis

47. **In keratomalacia which one is not found :** **WB 1998**
A. Corneal sensation
B. Inflammatory changes
C. Conjunctival kerosis
D. Melting & Liquefaction of cornea

48. **Epikeratophakia is used in :** **MAHE 1998**
A. Keratoconus B. Irregular cornea
C. Astigmatism D. Corneal scarring

49. **Keratitis sicca associated with :** **PGI 1990**
A. Sjogen's syndrome B. Gout
C. Lymphoproliferative D. Mucous secretion
E. Leukaemia

50. **In infective keratitis, which of the following is not done :** **Delhi 1998**
A. Tarsorrhaphy B. Keratoplasty
C. Paracentesis D. Chemical cauterisation

51. **Corneal ulceration is caused by injury to the —— cranial nerve.** **AIIMS 1983**
A. Third B. Fifth
C. Sixth D. Fourth

52. **The infant cornea attains the size of the adult cornea by which year :** **AIIMS 1983, 85**
A. 1 year B. 4 years
C. 8 years D. 9 years

53. **True statement about keratoglobus is :** **Delhi 1998**
A. Thinning of cornea
B. Increased visibility of corneal nerves
C. Fleischer's ring at the base of cornea
D. Cupping of the optic dis

54. **The colour of fluorescein staining in corneal ulcer is :** **AIIMS 1983**
A. Yellow B. Blue
C. Royal blue D. Green

55. **Corneal reflex is lost in the disease of :** **AI 1989**
A. Ophthalmia nerve
B. Ciliary ganglion
C. Supra-orbital nerve
D. Motor nucleus of 5th cranial nerve

56. **Dendritic ulcer is due to :** **AI 1988**
A. Herpes simplex B. Fungal infection
C. Syphilis D. Phlyctena

57. **Ophthalmia nodosa (granuloma in the sclera) is seen in :** **AI 1989**
A. Caterpillar hair in the eye
B. Granulomatous uveitis
C. Leprosy
D. None of the above

Ans.									
36. A	37. A	38. C	39. B	40. C	41. C	42. D	43. C	44. A	45. B
46. C	47. B	48. A	49. A	50. A	51. B	52. A	53. A	54. D	55. B
56. A	57. A								

58. **Sclera is weakest at : Delhi 1984, 86; DNB 1990, 92**
A. Limbus B. Posterior pole
C. Anterior pole D. Attachment of muscles

59. **In Keratoconus, the cone is situated at the : Orissa 1999**
A. Centre of the cornea
B. Just below the centre of the cornea
C. Just above the centre of the cornea
D. Either side of the corne

60. **Steroids are indicated in which type of herpes keratitis: JIPMER 2000**
A. Disciform keratitis B. Interstitial keratitis
C. Geographic ulcer D. Hypopyon ulcer

61. **Following are true about fungal keratitis except : AIIMS 1993; Delhi 2000**
A. Commonly blackish in colour
B. Satellite spots
C. Ciliary congestion
D. Hypopyon

62. **In Keratoconus, all are seen except : PGI 2000**
A. Munsun's sign
B. Thinning of cornea in center
C. Distortion of corneal reflex at center
D. Hypermetropic refractive error found

63. **Herpetic corneal ulcer is diagnosed by : UP 2000**
A. Geimsa stain B. ELISA
C. Cell culture/PCR D. Rose Bengal stain

64. **Branched septate hyphae found on corneal smear in a case of corneal ulcer is : AIIMS 2000**
A. Aspergillus B. Mucor
C. Candida D. Histoplasma

65. **In pseudomonas keratitis, used is all except : UP 1999**
A. Cephalosporin B. Polymyxin-B
C. Amikacin D. Piperacin

66. **Most common viral infection of the cornea is : Delhi 2001**
A. Herpes simplex B. Herpes zoster
C. Adenovirus D. Molluscum contagiosum

67. **Ocular symptom not seen in Herpes zoster ophthalmicus are except : AI 2001**
A. Oculomotor nerve involvement
B. Disciform keratitis
C. Anterior uveitis
D. Nummular keratitis

68. **A 30 years old male presents with a history of injury to the eye with a leaf 5 days ago and pain. Photophobia and redness of the eye for 2 days. What would be the most likely pathology : AIIMS 2002**
A. Anterior uveitis B. Conjunctivitis
C. Fungal corneal ulcer D. Corneal laceration

69. **A patient using contact lens develops corneal infection. Laboratory diagnosis of acanthomoeba keratitis was established. The following is the best drug for treatment : AI 2003**
A. Propamidine
B. Neosporine
C. Ketoconazole
D. Polyhexamethylene biguanide

70. **Corneal guttate is seen : MAHE 2003**
A. Fuch's endothelial dystrophy
B. Senile endothelial dystrophy
C. Secondary endothelial dystrophy
D. All of the above

71. **Cornea in blood stained is all except : CUPGME-2002**
A. Trauma
B. Subconjunctival haemorrhage
C. Low I.O.P
D. Perturis

72. **Which of the following will be the most important adjuvant therapy in a case of fungal corneal ulcer : AI 2004**
A. Atropine sulphate eye ointment
B. Dexamethasone eye drops
C. Pilocarpine eye drops
D. Lignocaine eye drops

73. **Enlarged corneal nerves may be seen in all of the following except : AI 2005**
A. Keratoconus
B. Herpes simplex keratitis
C. Leprosy
D. Neurofibromatosis

74. **All of following occur in herpes zoster ophthalmicus except : AIIMS 2011**
A. Pseudodendritic Keratitis
B. Anterior stromal Keratitis
C. Sclerokeratitis
D. Endothelitis

75. **Which of the following drug is currently used for the prophylaxis of non-infectious uveitis in LUMINATE programme : AIIMS 2011**
A. Cyclosporine B. Voclosporine
C. Methotrexate D. Infliximib

76. **What is the percentage of endothelial cell loss during Descemet's membrane stripping in automated penetrating Keratoplasty : AIIMS 2011**
A. 0-5 % B. 10-15%
C. 30-40% D. 50-60%

77. **Herpes zoster ophthalmicus least commonly involve ——————nerves : DNB 2011**
A. Facial B. Trigeminal
C. Lacrimal D. Nasociliary

Ans.									
58. D	59. B	60. B	61. A	62. C	63. D	64. A	65. B	66. A	67. A
68. C	69. A	70. A	71. C	72. A	73. B	74. C	75. B	76. C	77. B

78. **Carcumcorneal congestion is seen in following except :** DNB 2011

A. Anterior uveitis
B. Ac. congestive glaucoma
C. Steven Johnson syndrome
D. Moraxella infection

79. **Iris pearls are seen in :** DNB 2011

A. Leprosy
B. Eales disease
C. Sympathetic ophthalmia
D. High myopia

80. **Drug of choice in acute iridocyclitis :** DNB 2011

A. Oral steroid B. Topical steriods
C. Topical antibiotics D. Topical mydriatics

81. **Arf laser wavelength for LASIK surgery of cornea :** AI 2012

A. 126 B. 146
C. 193 D. 282

82. **Corneal lesion in a farmer showing feathery, vagetable matter is due to :** AI 2012

A. Diphtheria B. Fungal
C. Mechanical D. Mooren's ulcer

Ans. 78. D 79. A 80. D 81. C 82. B

EXPLANATIONS OF CORNEA & SCLERA

1. Ans. — C. If associated with glaucoma

2. Ans. — B. Pneumococci

   Common bacteria associated with corneal ulceration are Staphylococcus aureus, pseudomonas pyocyanea, streptococcus pneumoniae, E. coli, proteus, Klebsiella, N. gonorrhoea, N. meningitiis, C. diphtheriae.

3. Ans. — A. Calcerous degeneration

4. Ans. — D. Lacrimation

5. Ans. — C. Pneumococcus

6. Ans. — B. Streptococcus pneumoniae

   The characteristic hypopyon corneal ulcer caused by pneumococcus is called ulcus serpens. It has a tendency to creep over the cornea in a serpiginous fushion. The typical ulcus serpens is a greyish white or yellowish disc near the center of cornea.

7. Ans. — C. Action of the inflammatory fluid on the corneal endothelium.

8. Ans. — B. Polymorphonuclear leucocytes

9. Ans. — B. Endothelial dystrophy of Fuchs

10. Ans. — C. Pneumococcus

    It is customary to reserve the term hypopyon corneal ulcer for the characteristic ulcer caused by pneumococcus.

11. Ans. — C. Phlyctena

12. Ans. — A. Desmends

13. Ans. — C. Hypercellular stroma

14. Ans. — C. Leprosy

15. Ans. — B. Atropine

16. Ans. — C. Lens

    Voissius ring is a type of traumatic cataract. Sometimes a ring of brown granules of pigment with a faint opacity may form on the anterior lens capsule, just behind the pupillary margin.

17. Ans. — A. Retinitis pigmentosa

    Other causes are cataract and chronic simple glaucoma.

18. Ans. — A. Penetrating keratoplasty

    Keratoplasty or corneal graft is the ideal treatment.

19. Ans. — A. Leukoma adherent

20. Ans. — B. Watering

    Symptoms of a corneal ulcer are marked. During the progressive stage, there is lacrimation, photophobia, blepharospasm and pain, owing to the exposure of the terminal fibrils of the ophthalmic division of fifth nerve.

21. Ans. — A. Mycotic infection

    Pseudohypopyon is due to collection of tumor cells in anterior chamber may be seen in patients with retinoblastoma and malignant melanoma.

22. Ans. — C. Diptheria

23. Ans. — B. Anterior synychae

24. Ans. — C. Ciliary staphyloma

    Intercalary staphyloma occurs at the limbus immediately in front of the ciliary body. Etiology is the same as for ciliary staphyloma.

25. Ans. — C. Trigeminal nerve

26. Ans. — D. Is a narrow white ring of the sclera round the optic disc.

27. Ans. — E. None of the above

28. Ans. — D. None of the above

29. Ans. — B. Shallow anterior chamber

30. Ans. — A. Viral

    This is due to nerve involvement.

31. Ans. — D. Catarrhal conjunctivitis

32. Ans. — E. Keratocytes

33. Ans. — A. Measles

34. Ans. — B. Leber's optic neuropathy

35. Ans. — A. Hunter's disease

36. Ans. — A. Steroids accelerates recovery

Antibiotics, analgesics, and atropine are used. Local steroids are reserved for associated uveitis.

37. Ans. — A. I (iii) II (iv) III (ii) IV (i)

38. Ans. — C. Retinitis pigmentosa

39. Ans. — B. Substantia propria

40. Ans. — C. Macular

41. Ans. — C. 1.0

42. Ans. — D. Corneal graft

43. Ans. — C. Aspergillus

44. Ans. — A. Mooren's ulcer

45. Ans. — B. Epithelium

Epithelium tends to be raised into vesicles and bullae.

46. Ans. — C. Leprosy

47. Ans. — B. Inflammatory changes

48. Ans. — A. Keratoconus

In epikeratophakia, the lenticule prepared from the donor cornea is stitched over the surface of cornea after removing the epithelium. It is used for keratoconus.

49. Ans. — A. Sjogen's syndrome

50. Ans. — A. Tarsorrhaphy

51. Ans. — B. Fifth

52. Ans. — A. 1 year

53. Ans. — A. Thinning of cornea

In keratoglobus, there is thinning and excessive protrusion of cornea, which seems enlarged but its diameter is usually normal. It is hereditary bilateral, non-progressive and inherited as autosomal recessive trait.

54. Ans. — D. Green

55. Ans. — B. Ciliary ganglion

56. Ans. — A. Herpes simplex

It is usually caused by Herpes simplex forming an ulcer with branched appearance. It may occur at any age and is usual unilateral.

57. Ans. — A. Caterpillar hair in the eye

58. Ans. — D. Attachment of muscles

59. Ans. — B. Just below the centre of the cornea

60. Ans. — B. Interstitial keratitis

61. Ans. — A. Commonly blackish in colour

62. Ans. — C. Distortion of corneal reflex at center

In keratoconus, there is congenital weakness of cornea, though often it only menifests itself after puberty. Cone is just below the centre of cornea. Patient becomes myopic and contact lenses are more beneficial. If condition is progressive, corneal transplant may be needed.

63. Ans. — D. Rose Bengal stain

64. Ans. — A. Aspergillus

65. Ans. — B. Polymyxin-B

66. Ans. — A. Herpes simplex

67. Ans. — A. Oculomotor nerve involvement

68. Ans. — C. Fungal corneal ulcer

69. Ans. — A. Propamidine

- "Acanthamoeba keratitis can be a devastating infection if recognition is delayed & its occurrence is frequently associated with the wearing of soft contact lenses and the usual source of infection is the saline solution used to clean & store the lenses.
- When diagnosed early this chronic keratitis may be successfully treated with propamidine isethionate (Brolene).

70. Ans. — A. Fuch's endothelial dystrophy

71. Ans. — C. Low I.O.P

72. Ans. — A. Atropine sulphate eye ointment

Rx Fungal corneal ulcer

73. Ans. — B. Herpes simplex keratitis

74. Ans. — C. Sclerokeratitis

Herpes zoster ophthalmicus has following symptoms

Punctate epithelial keratitis	50%
Pseudodendritic keratitis	50%
Anterior stromal keratitis	40%
Endothelitis	34%
Serpiginous ulceration	7%
Scleral keratitis	1%

as sclerokeratitis is least commonly seen so answer of exclusion.

75. Ans. — B. Voclosporine

* The name of the drug is Luveniq [Voclosporin] which is calcineurin inhibitor and an immunomodulator.
* Voclosporin is a rationally designed novel calcineurin inhibitor used for prophylaxis of noninfectious uveitis.

76. Ans. — C. 30-40%

* DSAEK is a procedure which involves stripping of the diseased endothelium and descemet membrane with the donor graft which comprises of endothelium, descemet membrane and a small strip of posterior stroma.

This donor graft is harvested with a automated keratome. Since no sutures are required postop refractive error is least and the rehabilitation time is less compared to conventional penetrating keratoplasty [PK].The endothelial loss is more compared to PK and ranges from more than 20% to 25%.

77. Ans. — B. Trigeminal

Ophthalmic division is affected most often

78. Ans. — D. Moraxella infection

Moraxella causes angular conjunctivitis.

79. Ans. — A. Leprosy

Repeat Question. Iris pearls represent miliary lepromas.

80. Ans. — D. Topical mydriatisi

Repeat Question.. Scopolamine (25%) and atropine (1%) are best.

81. Ans. — C. 193

Wavelengths of lasers are

Excimer	Wavelength (nm)	Relative Power (mW)
Ar2	126	
Kr2	146	
Xe2	172 & 175	
Arf	193	60
KrF	248	100
XeBr	282	
XeCl	308	50
XeF	351	45
KrCl	222	25

82. Ans. — B. Fungal

Filamentary fungi in tropical and subtropic regions are fusorium and aspergillus and in temperate region, candida and aspergillus are the cause. Filamentary are aspergillus, fusarium, cephalosporium curvularia, penicillium whereas, yeast are candida, cryptococcus.

5

IMPORTANT TEXT OF CHAMBERS

ANTERIOR CHAMBER OF THE EYE

Boundaries of the anterior chamber

a. Anteriorly—The endothelial layer of the cornea.
b. Posteriorly—(i) At the angle by a part of the ciliary body. (ii) The whole of the iris. (iii) The lens in the pupillary aperture.

Normal depth of the anterior chamber—About **2.5 mm** in the central part.

Posterior Chamber

This is *triangular* space between the iris in front and the lens behind.

The boundaries of the posterior chamber are : (a) Anteriorly—Iris. (b) Posteriorly—The lens and the suspensory ligament. (c) Laterally—The ciliary body.

Aqueous Humour

Normally, the anterior and the posterior chambers are filled with a fluid called the aqueous humour.

1. ***Nature of the aqueous humour***—It is a slightly alkaline, clear, watery fluid with a density slightly higher than water. The volume of the aqueous in the anterior chamber is about **0.25 c.c.**, whereas that in the posterior chamber is about **0.06 c.c.**
2. ***Constituents of the aqueous humour***—It consists mainly of water and also of minute traces of all the diffusible constituents of the plasma. The protein content is negligible. But the sodium and the ascorbic acid are in a higher concentration than in plasma.
3. ***Source of the aqueous humour***—The chief source is from the ciliary process of the ciliary body and a very minute quantity from the vessels of the iris.
4. ***Mechanism of formation of the aqueous***—The exact mechanism is not known. But the present concept is that the aqueous is formed partly as a result of ultra-filtration through the capillary walls i.e., filtration under pressure and partly as a result of secretion by the ciliary processes, the latter process being more important. The mechanism of secretion also explain *higher sodium and ascorbic acid content* in the aqueous.
5. ***Functions of the aqueous humour***—It maintains the nutrition of the avascular structure like the cornea and the lens and also carries away their waste products. Also the clear aqueous in the anterior chamber takes part in the refraction of the light rays. But the more important function is that it helps to maintain a constant intra-ocular pressure.
6. ***Rate of flow of aqueous humour***—Depending upon the technique employed the rate of flow of the aqueous humour has been found to vary from **1 to 5 cu mm per minute.**

NARROW ANTERIOR CHAMBER ANGLE (May be Capable of Angle Closure Glaucoma)

1. Normal variation
2. Predisposition to angle closure
3. Anterior dislocation of the lens
4. Hyperopia
5. Spherophakia and microcornea

6. Post-operative intraocular operation with leaking wound
7. Choroidal detachment
8. Pupillary block
9. Loss of aqueous from perforating ulcer, corneal wound, or staphyloma
10. Intumescent senile cataract
11. Traumatic cataract that fluffs-up
12. Primary hyperplastic primary vitreous
13. Peripheral anterior synechiae
14. Posterior entrapment of aqueous humor (malignant glaucoma of ciliary-block glaucoma)
15. Drugs including; acetazolamide, acetylcholine, alpha-chymotrypsin, demecarium, dichlorphenamide, echothiophate, edrophonium, ethoxzolamide, isoflurophatc, methazolamide, neostigmine, physostigmine, pilocarpine, sulfacetamide, sulfachlorpyridazine, sulfadiazine, sulfadimethoxine, sulfamerazine, sulfameter, sulfamethizole, sulfamethoxazole, sulfamethoxypyridazine, sulfanilamide, sulfaphenazole, sulfisoxazole

MCQ's OF CHAMBERS

What is important in Chambers

Anterior and posterior, Mechanism of formation of aqueous

1. **Flat anterior chamber may result due to :** **AIIMS 1982**
   A. Occlusion by pupil by exudates
   B. Seclusio pupillae
   C. Leakage after cataract operation
   D. Acute congestive glaucoma
   E. Any of the above

2. **In uremic amaurosis :** **Bihar 1998**
   A. Pupil is constricted
   B. Pupil is dilated and unresponsive to light
   C. Pupil is dilated and responsive to light
   D. Pupil dilates in response to light

3. **Normal intraocular pressure is :** **Delhi 1987**
   A. 0-5 mm Hg B. 6-10 mm Hg
   C. 11-15 mm Hg D. 16-12 mm Hg

4. **Rate of absorption (mL/min) of Aqueous humour is :** **MAHE 1999**
   A. 1.0 B. 2.0
   C. 3.0 D. 4.0

5. **Shallow anterior chamber is seen in :** **Orissa 1999**
   A. High myopia
   B. Aphakia
   C. High hypermetropria
   D. All of the above conditions

6. **The components of the normal vitreous include following except :** **AIIMS 1983**
   A. Collagen B. N-acetyl glycosamine
   C. Calcium salts D. Hyaluronic acid
   E. Ascorbat

7. **The following are important in the production and/or release of aqueous except :** **PGI 1983**
   A. Parasympathetic nerves
   B. Pigmented epithelium
   C. Ultrafiltration and diffusion
   D. Adenylate cyclase
   E. Carbonic anhydrase

8. **Floaters can be seen in following except :** **AIIMS 1995, 97**
   A. Ac congestive glaucoma
   B. Uveitis
   C. Retinal detachment
   D. Vitreous haemorrhage

9. **Angle of anterior chamber is studied with:** **Delhi 1992**
   A. Indirect ophthalmoscopy
   B. Gonioscopy
   C. Retinopathy
   D. Amblyoscope

10. **Lacrimal sac :** **TNPSC 1997**
    A. It is a muscular bag
    B. Situated in the lacrimal groove
    C. Upper end is blind
    D. Lower end is tubular

11. **Features of asteriod bodies in the vitreous include:** **AIIMS 1982**
    A. Clinically innocous
    B. Composed of crystalline spherical bodies
    C. Consist of calcium crystals
    D. Usually bilateral
    E. All of the above

12. **Pupils are mid dilated and fixed in :** **AIIMS 1997**
    A. Acute congestive glaucoma
    B. Chronic congestive glaucoma
    C. Open angle glaucoma
    D. Closed angle glaucoma

Ans.	1. E	2. C	3. D	4. B	5. C	6. C	7. B	8. B	9. B	10. C
	11. E	12. A								

13. **Aqueous humour formation occurs by all means, except:** **AMU 1987; DNB 1990**
A. Ultrafiltration B. Active secretion
C. Passive diffusion D. Denovo synthesis

14. **Aqueous humour :** **TNPSC 1997**
A. Is viscous fluid
B. Fills anterior and posterior chambers
C. Is a dialysate from the capillaries
D. Poured into the posterior chamber

15. **Raised LHD levels in Aqueous is seen in :** **AI 2009**
A. Galactosemia
B. Glaucoma
C. Hemangioblastoma
D. Retinoblastoma

16. **Jet black pupil, deep anterior chamber with scar as limbus with 6/6 vision with lens, diagnosis is :** **AI 2012**
A. Akhakia
B. Pseudophakia
C. Posterior dislocation of lens
D. Hypermetropia

17. **White pupillary reflex, retina totally normal, chalky white optic disc. Which is cause :** **AI 2012**
A. Diabetic retinopathy
B. Primary optic neuritis
C. Traumatic lens dislocation
D. Trachoma

18. **Dilator pupillae is supplied by : AIIMS 2011, AI 2012**
A. Postganglionic sympathetic from cervical plexus
B. Preganglionic sympathetic from cervical plexus
C. III Nerve
D. Postganglionic sympathetic fibres from V nerve.

Ans. 13. D 14. B 15. D 16. C 17. B 18. A

EXPLANATIONS OF CHAMBERS

1. Ans. — E. Any of the above
2. Ans. — C. Pupil is dilated and responsive to light
3. Ans. — D. 16-12 mm Hg

   Normal IOP is 10 to 21 mmHg (mean 16± 2-5 mmHg).
4. Ans. — B. 2.0
5. Ans. — C. High hypermetropria
6. Ans. — C. Calcium salts
7. Ans. — B. Pigmented epithelium
8. Ans. — B. Uveitis
9. Ans. — B. Gonioscopy

   Gonioscopy is used for biomicroscopic examination of angle of anterior chamber. Two types of goniolens are used— (i) Indirect goniolens provides a mirror image of the opposite angle e.g. Goldmann and the Zeiss goniolens (ii) Direct goniolens - provides a direct view of the angle. Koeppe goniolens is the most popular type.
10. Ans. — C. Upper end is blind
11. Ans. — E. All of the above
12. Ans. — A. Acute congestive glaucoma
13. Ans. — D. Denovo synthesis

    Aqueous humour is a clear watery fluid filling the anterior chamber (0.25 ml) and posterior chamber (0.06ml) of the eyeball. Ultrafiltration and diffusion are dependent on the level of B.P. in ciliary capillaries, the plasma osmotic pressure and the level of IOP.
14. Ans. — B. Fills anterior and posterior chambers
15. Ans. — D. Retinoblastoma
    * Inheritance—Ad, but only 6% cases are familial
    * Familial cases have early onset, bilateral involvement an are predisposed to develop second non ocular malignancy including pinealoblastoma and osteogenic sarcoma
    * B/L Retinoblastoma with pinealo-blastoma is termed as trilateral retino-blastoma
    * The specific area corresponding to retinoblastoma gene was identified on 14 band, on long arm of chromosome 13—13 q 14
16. Ans. — C. Posterior dislocation of lens

    These signs indicate dislocation of lens.
17. Ans. — B. Primary optic neuritis

    Pain in affected eye, sudden loss of vision, and decrease in color (red) vision, swollen optic nerve but nerve normal indicates optic neuritis. Multiple sclerosis is a cause.
18. Ans. — A. Postganglionic sympathetic from cervical plexus

    These nerves act by releasing noradrenaline which acts on alpha 1 receptors. Supply is from T_2 sympathetic chain ganglion through axons along ciliary arteries.

DM/MCh ENTRANCE EXAMINATION SERIES

Contains **Important Text, Original Solved MCQ's** and their **explanations** for following

DM/MCh Entrance Examinations :-

- DM Neurology & MCh Neurosurgery
- DM Cardiology & MCh Cardiothoracic surgery
- DM Gastroenterology and MCh Gastrosurgery
- DM Nephrology & MCh Urosurgery
- MCh Burns & Plastic Surgery
- MCh Pediatric Surgery
- DM Endocrinology
- DM Pulmonary Medicine
- DM Neonatology
- A useful book for DM/MCh/DNB Examinations
- Edited by **Dr. M.S. Bhatia** (MD, Wip WPA), DNB and **Dr. Nirmaljit Kaur** (MD) experienced editors, examiners & paper setters.

Keep your knowledge uptodate with this new series from:

CBS Publishers & Distributors Pvt. Ltd.

NEW DELHI • BANGALORE • PUNE • CHENNAI • COCHIN (INDIA)

6

IMPORTANT TEXT OF UVEAL TRACT

RUBEOSIS IRIDIS (Neovascularization [Newly Formed Blood Vessles] on iris)

= Most Important

1. **Proximal vascular diseases**
   A. Aortic arch syndrome (pulseless disease; Takayasu syndrome).
   B. Carotid-cavernous fistula carotid artery syn drome).
   C. Carotid ligation
   D. Carotid occlusive disease
   E. Cranial arteritis syndrome (giant-cell arteritis)
2. **Ocular vascular diseases**
   * A. Central retinal artery thrombosis
   * B. Central retinal vein thrombosis
   C. Long posterior ciliary artery occlusion
   D. Reversed flow through the ophthalmic artery
3. **Retinal diseases**
   A. Coats disease (retinal telangiectasia)
   * B. Diabetes mellitus
   C. Eales disease (periphlebitis)
   D. Glaucoma, chronic
   E. Melanoma of choroid
   F. Norrie disease (oligophrenia-microphthalmos syndrome)
   G. Persistent hyperplastic primary vitreous
   H. Retinal detachment
   I. Retinal hemangioma
   J. Retinoblastoma
   K. Retrolental fibroplasia
   L. Sickle cell disease (Herrick syndrome)
4. **Iris tumors**
   A. Hemangioma
   B. Melanoma
   C. Metastatic carcinoma
5. **Post-inflammatory**
   A. Argon laser coreoplasty
   B. Exfoliation syndrome
   C. Fibrinoid syndrome
   D. Fungal endophthalmitis
   E. Iris neovascularization with pseudoexfoliation
   F. Radiation
   G. Retinal detachment operation
   H. Uveitis, chronic
6. **Vascular tuffs at the pupillary margin**
   A. Cataract
   B. Diabetes mellitus
   C. Myotonic dystrophy syndrome (myotonia atrophica syndrome).
   D. Ocular hypotony
   E. Respiratory failure

INTRAOCULAR CALCIFICATIONS

1. Choroidal osteoma
2. Facial nevus of Jadassohn (linear sebaceous nevus syndrome).
3. Intraocular calcifications
   A. Congenital deformity
   B. Recurrent iritis and keratitis
   C. Retinal detachment
   D. Trauma (perforating, non-perforating, or surgical).
4. Intraocular sarcoma
5. Retinoblastoma
6. Retrolental fibroplasia
7. Sites of intraocular calcification
   A. Calcific emboli of retinal and ciliary arteries
   B. Cyclitic membrane
   C. Lens
   D. Peripapillary choroid
   E. Posterior pole to ora serrata in region of choroid and pigment epithelium
   F. Retina
   G. Vitreous

PHTHISIS BULBI (Degenerative Shrinkage of Eyeball with Hypotony)

1. Following cataract surgery, especially with rubella syndrome (German measles).
2. Panophthalmitis
3. Severe ocular injury with loss of tissue.
4. Severe uveitis
5. Sympathetic ophthalmia
6. Tumor, such as retinoblastoma or malignant melanoma.

ANGIOID STREAKS (Ruptures of Bruch Membrane Characterized Ophthalmoscopically by Brownish Lines Surrounding the Disc and Radiating toward the Periphery)

1. Acromegaly
2. Cardiovascular disease with hypertension
3. Cooley anemia
4. Diffuse lipomatosis
5. Dwarfism
6. Epilepsy
7. Facial angiomatosis
8. Fibrodysplasia hyperelastica (Ehlers-Danlos syndrome).
9. Francois dyscephalic syndrome (Hallermann-Streff syndrome).
10. Lead poisoning
11. Ocular melanocytosis
12. Osteitis deformans (Paget's disease)
13. Pituitary tumor
14. Previous choroidal detachment
15. Pseudoxanthoma elasticum (Gronblad-Strandberg syndrome).
16. Senile (actinic) elastosis of the skin
17. Sickle cell disease (Herrick syndrome)
18. Thrombocytopenic purpura

PSEUDODETACHMENT OF VITREOUS (Conditions Simulating Detachment of Vitreous)

1. Enormous cavity in the vitreous body with a relatively thin posterior wall.
2. Membranous formations within the vitreous associated with uveitis and haemorrhage.
3. Outline of the ascending portion of Cloquet canal just anterior to the disc.

ANTERIOR VITREOUS DETACHMENT (Anterior Vitreous May Be Separated from Posterior Lens or Posterior Zonular Fibers)

1. Retrolenticular—usually caused by vitreous shrinkage
   - A. Trauma
   - B. Haemorrhage
   - C. Senescence
   - D. Inflammation
   - E. Retinal detachment
2. Retrozonular
   - A. Vitreous shrinkage
   - B. Ciliary body tumor
   - C. Blood
   - D. Exudate
3. Retrolenticular and retrozonular combined occurs with rupture of the hyaloideocapsular ligament

POSTERIOR VITREOUS DETACHMENT

1. Complete posterior detachment

A. Simple detachment—occurs in young persons
   - (i) Exudate from chorioretinitic focus.
   - (ii) Hemorrhage between the vitreous and the retina.
   - (iii) Retraction of the cortical vitreous caused by exudate within the vitreous.
   - (iv) Vitreous haemorrhage in a young individual with vitreous shrinking because of thrombosis of central retinal vein, retinitis proliferans, central serous retinopathy, or trauma.

B. Complete posterior detachment with collapse
   - (i) Senescence changes are primary cause
   - (ii) Uveitis
   - (iii) Trauma
   - (iv) Haemorrhage
   - (v) Sodium hyaluronate

C. Funnel-shapped posterior detachment
   - (i) Perforating injuries of globe
   - (ii) Retinitis proliferans
   - (iii) Massive vitreous detachment

D. Atypical complete posterior detachment—Residual adherence of vitreous to a peripheral retinal area :
   - (i) Focus of chorioretinitis
   - (ii) Following cataract extraction with loss of vitreous.
   - (iii) Following perforating wounds

2. Partial posterior detachment (unusual).

A. Superior detachment—Primarily a senescence change, generally forerunner of posterior vitreous detachment with collapse.

B. Partial posterior detachment (not infrequent)
   (i) Preretinal haemorrhage
   (ii) Retinitis proliferans
C. Partial lateral or partial inferior detachment
   (i) Focus of choroiditis
   (ii) Circumscribed retinal periphlebitis
   (iii) Intraocular foreign body

BEADS IN VITREOUS (Snowballs in Vitreous)

1. African eye-worm disease (Iloiasis)
2. Amyloidosis (Lubarsch-Pick syndrome)
3. Bang disease (brucellosis)
4. Bechet syndrome (dermatostomato-ophthalmic syndrome)
5. Criswick-Schepens syndrome (familial exudative vitreoretinopathy)
6. Hemophilus influenzae
7. Irvine syndrome
8. Jacobsen-Brodwall syndrome
9. Japanese river fever (typhus)
10. Oculo-oto-ororenoerythropoietic disease
11. Pars planitis
12. Retinoblastoma
13. Sarcoid (Schaumann syndrome)
14. Severe uveitis
15. Toxic lens syndrome
16. Vogt-Koyanagi-Harada syndrome (uveitis-vitiligo-alopecia-poliosis syndrome)

VITREOUS LIQUEFACTION

1. Myopia
2. Peripheral uveitis
3. Retinitis pigmentosa
4. Spontaneous
5. Trauma
6. With aging
7. With vitreous traction as Wagner disease

MCQ's OF UVEAL TRACT

What is important in Uveal Tract

Pupil (Reflexes), Argyl-Robertson Pupil (Classical & reverse type), Hutchison's pupil, Causes of abnormalities (unilateral/bilateral, miosis/mydriasis), Iridocyclitis (D/D of red Eye), Vitreous

1. **Uveal tuberculosis should be suspected in the following : AMU 1986, 90**
   A. Periphlebitis retinae
   B. Iris nodules proved not to be sarcoidosis
   C. Chronic granulomatous uveitis
   D. Spreading choroiditis along with episcleritis
   E. All of the above
2. **Marcus Gunn Pupil indicates disease of : AMU 1989, 93**
   A. Lens B. Sclera
   C. Retina D. Optic nerve
3. **A severe iridocyclitis characterised by the formation of granulomatous lesion (ophthalmia nodosa) occurs in : MP 1998**
   A. Chalicosis
   B. Granulomatous uveitis
   C. Siderosis bulbi
   D. Penetration of caterpillar hair inside the eye
4. **In complete albinism the colour of iris is : TN 1989, 95**
   A. White B. Black
   C. Pink D. Blue
   E. Green
5. **Essential atrophy of the choroid is a consequence of disordered metabolism of : AIIMS 1990; Bihar 1998**
   A. Phenylalanine B. Cysteine
   C. Ornithine D. Arginine
6. **One of the following is an absolute contraindication in acute anterior uveitis : AI 1995, 99**
   A. Timolol B. Atropine
   C. Steroids D. Cyclopentolate
7. **To prevent sympathetic ophthalmia, it is best to remove the injured eye before : Karnataka 1998**
   A. One month after the accident
   B. Nine days after the accident
   C. Two weeks after the accident
   D. Three days after the accident
8. **'Mutton-fat' precipitates in slit lamp examination are seen in : TN 1996**
   A. Granulomatous iridocyclitis
   B. Choroiditis
   C. Non-Granulomatous iridocyclitis
   D. Vitreous haemorrhage
9. **In anterior uveitis, anterior chamber is : PGI 1982; AIIMS 1984;**
   A. Narrow
   B. Deep
   C. Normal
   D. Narrow and later on becomes deep
10. **The commonest parasitic cause of uveitis is : AIIMS 1984, 89**
    A. Toxoplasma B. Amoebiasis
    C. Taenia solium D. Oncocercosis
11. **All of the statements are true about band keratopathy except : Rajasthan 1994**
    A. Lies in inter-palpebral area.
    B. Seen in old Blind Shrunken eyes due to defective nutrition & Exposure.
    C. Does not cause chronic uveitis.
    D. Is due to hyaline infiltration of the superfical parts of stroma followed by deposition of calcerous salts (EDTA dissolvable).
12. **Following injury to exciting eye, sympathetic ophthalmitis begins : WB 1996; UPSC 1997**
    A. In 4 to 6 days B. In 4 to 6 weeks
    C. In 8 to 12 weeks D. After 12 weeks
13. **The most diagnostic sign of anterior uveitis is : AIIMS 1986, 87; Delhi 1989**
    A. Aqueous flare
    B. Keratitic precipitates
    C. Constriction of pupil
    D. Raised intra-ocular tension

Ans. 1. E 2. D 3. D 4. C 5. C 6. A 7. C 8. A 9. A 10. A 11. C 12. B 13. B

14. **A child having healed central choroiditis in both the eyes should be investigated for : AIIMS 1986; Rajasthan 1998**
A. Histoplasma B. Toxoplasma
C. Entamoeba histolytica D. Tuberculosis

15. **Acute intermittent conjunctivitis or anterior uveitis or keratitis is seen in : AIIMS 1987**
A. Rhuematoid arthritis
B. Systemic lupus erythematosus
C. Reiter's syndrome
D. Sjogren's syndrome

16. **The commonest cause of white pupil in children is : PGI 1987**
A. Persistent papillary membrane
B. Uveitis
C. Endophthalmitis
D. Cataract
E. Retinoblastoma

17. **All of the following cause panuveitis except : Delhi 1998**
A. Ankylosing spondylitis
B. Toxoplasmosis
C. Sarcoidosis
D. Sympathetic ophthalmitis

18. **Most common cause of anterior uveitis is : AIIMS 1998**
A. Ankylosing spondylitis B. Rheumatoid arthritis
C. Behcet's syndrome D. Sarcoidosis

19. **Uveitis in Rheumatoid arthritis is seen in——type. AIIMS 1997**
A. Systemic B. Pauciarticular
C. JRA + D. JRA -ve

20. **Amaurotic cat's eye reflex is seen in : PGI 1984**
A. Papilloedema B. Retinoblastoma
C. Papillitis D. Retinitis

21. **Of the following which is the shortest acting mydriatic : AIIMS 1992**
A. Tropicamide B. Homatropine
C. Cyclopentolate D. Atropine

22. **'D' shaped pupil is seen in : JIPMER 1993**
A. Iridocyclitis B. Iridodialysis
C. Glaucoma D. Dislocation of lens

23. **Uveitis is characterized by all except : TN 1993; PGI 2000**
A. Mucopurulent discharge
B. Small pupils
C. Moderate pain
D. Marked tenderness

24. **Which one of the following is not anomaly of the pupil : DNB 1991**
A. Anosocoria B. Iridodiastasis
C. Corectopia D. Dyscoria
E. Polycoria

25. **Dalen fuch's nodules are seen in : Delhi 1993**
A. Sympathetic ophthalmia
B. Phithisis bulbi
C. Absolute glaucoma
D. Psudoxanthoma - elasticum

26. **Small pupils are seen in : AP 1991**
A. Argyll Robertson pupil
B. Adie pupil
C. IIIrd nerve palsy
D. Mydriatric drops instillation

27. **There is no pupillary abnormality in IIIrd cranial nerve palsy if the patient has : PGI 1984**
A. Sustained trauma
B. Anterior cerebral artery aneurysm
C. Diabetes mellitus
D. Sarcoidosis
E. Tuberculosis

28. **The most frequent bacterial agent causing non-granulomatous uveitis is : Delhi 1988**
A. Staphylococcus B. Streptococcus
C. Pneumococcus D. Influenza bacillus

29. **Recurrent attacks of non-granulomatous uveitis lead to : Delhi 1984**
A. Secondary cataract
B. Band keratopathy
C. Persistent extensive synechiae
D. Phthisis bulbi
E. All of the above

30. **Number of plications around the circumference of ciliary body seen macroscopically is about : AIIMS 1983**
A. 25 B. 40
C. 55 D. 70
E. 85

31. **Ill-sustained pupillary reaction is seen in : AIIMS 1986**
A. Chronic simple glaucoma
B. Optic neuritis
C. Iritis
D. Papilloedema
E. None of the above

32. **Central scotoma is seen in : Bihar 1989**
A. Retrobulbar neuritis B. Chronic glaucoma
C. Nuclear cataract D. Corneal opacitis

33. **Physiological tone of ciliary muscle is about : AMU 1984**
A. Three diopters B. Four diopters
C. One diopter D. 2.5 diopter
E. 3.5 diopter

Ans.	14. B	15. C	16. E	17. A	18. A	19. B	20. B	21. A	22. B	23. A
	24. B	25. A	26. A	27. C	28. B	29. E	30. D	31. B	32. A	33. C

34. Diagnostic features of malignant melanoma of the iris include all except : PGI 1986
A. Blood vessels in the tumor
B. Glaucoma
C. Implantation growth in the iris
D. Acquired freckles on the iris
E. None of the above

35. Bilateral facial palsy and posterior uveitis of recent onset is likely to be due to which of the following : AIIMS 1983; UPSC 1987
A. Motor neurone disease B. Melkerson's syndrome
C. Moebius' syndrome D. Sarcoidosis
E. Disseminated sclerosis

36. During accommodation all the following changes occur except : AIIMS 1983
A. Pupil contracts
B. Anterior chamber shallows
C. Lens becomes thinner
D. Anterior and posterior surface of the lens become convex
E. Lens sinks down

37. A patient under treatment for Graves disease (diffuse toxic goitre) has unilateral exophthalmos and one pupil larger than the other. Which of the following is the most likely cause for the anisocoria : AMU 1985; AIIMS 1986
A. Adie's pupil B. Horner's syndrome
C. Third nerve palsy D. Thyrotoxic myopathy
E. Topical medication

38. All are true about heredomacular degeneration, except : AIIMS 1983, 87, 91
A. The neuroepithelium is normal
B. The condition appears at puberty
C. The electroetinogram is normal
D. Inheritance is usually recessive

39. Features of iritis include all of the following, except : BHU 1986; JIPMER 1993
A. Small pupil
B. Normal pupilary reaction
C. Cilliary congestion
D. Aqueous flare
E. Loss of iris pattern

40. Non granulomatous uveitis is characterised histological by all of the following, except : Karnataka 1989
A. Neovascularization
B. Nodules of plasma cells
C. Nodules of lymphocytes
D. Cellular infiltration of iris

41. Commonest cause of vitreous haemorrhage in a young adult is : Karnataka 1989
A. Diabetes
B. Trauma
C. Periphlebitis retinae
D. Central retinal vein occlusion

42. All of the following statements about vitreous detachment are true except : MAHE 1996
A. It is a common change in middle age.
B. It is usually of no pathological significance.
C. It may initiate a retinal detachment.
D. It requires surgical replacement.

43. In a case with anterior uveitis, which of the following X-ray is useful in determining the etiology : Delhi 1994
A. Sacroiliac joint B. Dental checkup
C. X-ray chest D. Mantoux reaction

44. Typical coloboma of the iris is situated : AIIMS 1987
A. Superiorly B. Inferiorly
C. Superio-nasally D. Inferio-nasally

45. Subacute uveitis with glaucoma which drug shou!d not be given : AIIMS 1985
A. Pilocarpine B. Timolol
C. Ectohiopate D. Atropine

46. Synechiae in iris bombe are : AI 1994, 97, 99
A. Ring synechiae B. Total synechiae
C. Gonio synechiae D. All of the above

47. All of the following statements about the treatment of acute anterior uveitis are true except : MAHE 1996
A. Mydriasis is important.
B. Steroids should be avoided.
C. It is usually not necessary to admit the patient to the hospital.
D. Investigations for systemic disease are often negative.

48. A young female with fibrinous uveitis, next investigation is : PGI 1995
A. Chest X-ray B. X-ray sacroiliac joint
C. Mantoux test D. ESR

49. The earliest feature of anterior uveitis includes : PGI 1987
A. Keratic precipitates B. Hypopyon
C. Posterior synechiae D. Aqueous flare

50. The state of the pupil during sleep is : AIIMS 1989
A. Constricted B. Dilated
C. Normal size D. None of the above

Ans. 34. E 35. D 36. C 37. E 38. A 39. B 40. A 41. B 42. D 43. A
44. D 45. A 46. A 47. B 48. B 49. D 50. A 51. C

51. Which of the following statement is true : MAHE 1996

A. The uvea is not pigmented.
B. Iridocyclitis means recurrent inflammation of the iris.
C. The terms iridocyclitis and anterior uveitis are synonymous..
D. The iris is entirely derived from the mesoderm.

52. Early feature of sympathetic ophthalmia is : AI 1997

A. Aqueous flare B. RL flare
C. Mydriasis D. Miosis

53. Dilated pupil is seen in all of the following except : AP 1990

A. Pontine haemorrhage B. Optic trophy
C. Acute glaucoma D. Papillitis

54. In gouty iritis following are found except : PGI 1981

A. Granulomatous iritis
B. Non-granulomatous iritis
C. Associated scleritis
D. Frequently recovery

55. Vitreous hemorrhage is not seen in : Kerala 1996

A. Hypertension B. Eale's disease
C. Trauma D. DM
E. Vitreous degeneration

56. Asteroid hyalitis is : PGI 1983

A. Clinically symptomless
B. Presents bilaterally in three fourth of cases
C. Composed of crystalline spherical bodies
D. All of the above

57. In a frightened man, the pupil shall : AI 1988

A. Dilate
B. First dilate and then constrict
C. Constrict
D. Remain unaltered

58. Choroiditis due to separation of rods & cones is characterized by : Kerala 1998

A. Micropsia
B. Macropsia
C. Irregularity of surface seen
D. All of the above

59. Drug of choice for Acute Iridocylitis is : Delhi 1992; AIIMS 1992, 93

A. Acetazolamide B. Atropine
C. Antibiotics D. Aspirit

60. Commonest cause of persistent pupillary membrane is : DNB 1989

A. Fetal Iritis
B. Hereditary
C. Physiologic
D. Use of oxygen therapy in premature

61. Iridodialysis is : PGI 1982, 86, 87, 88

A. Iris is broken from ciliary body
B. Hole in iris
C. Tremulousness of iris
D. All of the above

62. Which of the following is not a cause of fixed dilated pupil : Delhi 1982; PGI 1984; ESI 1985, 90

A. Corneal ulcer
B. Iridocyclitis
C. Acute congestive glaucoma
D. Atropine ointment

63. True about heterochrome iritis is : Delhi 1989

A. Hyperpigmented iris
B. Hypopigmented iris
C. Coarse keratic precipitates
D. Glaucoma

64. Examination of vitreous is best done by : AIIMS 1986, 89

A. Direct ophthalmoscope
B. Indirect ophthalmoscope
C. Slit lamp with contact lens
D. Uveitis

65. Pupillary reflex is lost in : Delhi 1986

A. Optic neuritis B. Glaucoma
C. Iridocyclitis D. Adie pupil

66. Pin point pupil is caused by : Delhi 1990

A. Organophosphorus B. Alcohol
C. Barbiturates D. Opiates

67. Organism most commonly isolated from the vitreous following endophthalmitis developing 9 days after cataract surgery is : Delhi 1997

A. Staph. epidermidis B. Bacillus subtilis
C. Pseudo. pyocyanea D. Strep. viridans

68. Vitreous opacities may be due to : PGI 1987, 90

A. Herpetic keratouveitis B. Posterior uvetitis
C. Hyaloid asteroides D. High myopia

69. Commonest cause of vitreous haemorrhage is : PGI 1983, 84

A. Diabetes B. Hypertension
C. Lens extraction D. Trauma

70. Pupil size is increased in : Delhi 1988

A. Sleep B. Anxiety
C. Near accommodation D. Eserine instillation

71. Atropine sulphate 1% drop or ointment must be used to apically in : Orissa 1999

A. Acute conjuctivitis
B. Chronic conjuctivitis
C. Iritis
D. Acute congestive glaucoma

Ans.									
52. A	53. A	54. A	55. E	56. D	57. A	58. D	59. B	60. D	61. A
62. A	63. B	64. C	65. D	66. D	67. C	68. D	69. D	70. B	71. C
72. C	73. D								

72. In Iridocyclitis, not seen in : Delhi 1988
A. KP (Keratic Precipitates)
B. Turbid aqueous
C. Miosis
D. Circumcorneal congestion

73. Commonest cause of posterior staphyloma is : AIIMS 1987
A. Glaucoma B. Retinal detachment
C. Iridocyclitis D. High myopia

74. Iridocyclitis is most commonly seen in : Delhi 1999
A. Pauciarticular juvenile rheumatoid arthritis (JRA)
B. Multiarticular JRA
C. Systemic JRA
D. None of the above

75. Rubeosis iridis is not seen in : PGI 1999
A. CRVO B. CRAO
C. Diabetic retinopathy D. Neovascularization

76. Snowbanking is typically seen in : PGI 1999
A. Pars planitis B. Endophthalmitis
C. Coat's disease D. Eale's disease

77. Following is a part of uvea except : Kerala 1999
A. Bowman's membrane B. Iris
C. Ciliary body D. Choroid

78. Nodule on iris is seen in all except : UP 1999
A. Tuberculosis B. Sarcoidosis
C. Neurofibromatosis D. Still's disease

79. Chronic uveitis is seen in all except : UP 1999
A. Sarcoidosis B. Pauciarticular RA
C. Brucellosis D. Herpetic uveitis

80. Iris is thinnest at : UP 1999, 2001
A. Collarette B. Pupil margin
C. Base (Root) D. Ciliary zone

81. In which of the following conditions, iridectomy is indicated : Kerala 2000, 2003
A. Prolapsed Iris
B. Closed angle glaucoma
C. As part of cataract extraction
D. Threatening ring synechia
E. All of the above

82. 25-years-old Kalloo, presents with one day history of pain and redness associated with watering from his left eye. This was associated with intolerance to light. What is the most probable diagnosis : AI 2000
A. Acute anterior uveitis
B. Acute posterior uveitis
C. Epidemic keratoconjunctivitis
D. Keratitis

83. Koeppe's & Busca's nodules are characteristic of : JIPMER 2002
A. Granulomatous uveitis
B. Non-granulomatous uveitis
C. Residual uveitis
D. Recurrent uveitis

84. All the following are true regarding acute anterior uveitis in Ankylosing spondylitis except : SGPGI 2002, 2004
A. More common in females.
B. Recurrent attacks occur.
C. Fibrous reaction in anterior chamber.
D. Narrowing of joint spaces and sclerosis of sacroiliac joint.

85. Iridocorneal endothelial syndrome is associated with : AIIMS 2008
A. Progressive atrophy of iris stroma
B. Bilateral stromal edema of iris & cornea
C. Deposition of collagen in Descemet's membrane
D. Deposition of glycosaminoglycan in Descemet's membrane

86. True about Uveal effusion syndrome is all except : AI 2009
A. Due to defect in sclera
B. Choroido-retinal detachment
C. Scleritis
D. Myopia

87. Non-pigmented epithelium of ciliary body : DNB 2011
A. Continuation of pigmentary epithelium
B. Contintuation of Bruch's membrane of choroid
C. Continuation of ora serrata
D. None of the above

Ans. 74. A	75. B	76. A	77. A	78. D	79. D	80. C	81. E	82. A	83. A
84. A	85. A	86. D	87. A						

EXPLANATIONS OF UVEAL TRACT

1. Ans.— E. All of the above
2. Ans.— D. Optic nerve

   Marcus Gunn pupil is the parodoxical response of a pupil to light in the presence of a relative afferent pathway defect (RAPD). It is tested by swinging flash light test.
3. Ans.— D. Penetration of caterpillar hair inside the eye.
4. Ans.— C. Pink
5. Ans.— C. Ornithine
6. Ans.— A. Timolol

   It is a parasympathomimetic mydriatic and is contraindicated.
7. Ans.— C. Two weeks after the accident
8. Ans.— A. Granulomatous iridocyclitis
9. Ans.— A. Narrow
10. Ans.— A. Toxoplasma

    Congenital toxoplasmosis is characterized by a triad- convulsion, chorioretinitis and intracranial calcification. When pregnant females catch the disease about 49% infants are born with the disease (active or inactive). Toxocara is another intestinal round worm causing endophthalmitis.
11. Ans.— C. Does not cause chronic uveitis
12. Ans.— B. In 4 to 6 weeks
13. Ans.— B. Keratitic precipitates
14. Ans.— B. Toxoplasma
15. Ans.— C. Reiter's syndrome
16. Ans.— E. Retinoblastoma
17. Ans.— A. Ankylosing spondylitis
18. Ans.— A. Ankylosing spondylitis

    About 50% of patients with acute anterior uveitis passess HLA-B27. Uveitis is associated with ankylosing spondylitis or Reiter's syndrome in a high proportion of men.
19. Ans.— B. Pauciarticular
20. Ans.— B. Retinoblastoma
21. Ans.— A. Tropicamide
22. Ans.— B. Iridodialysis
23. Ans.— A. Mucopurulent discharge
24. Ans.— B. Iridodiastasis
25. Ans.— A. Sympathetic ophthalmia

    Dalen-Fuchs nodules are formed due to proliferation of the pigment epithelium (of the iris, ciliary body and choroid) associated with invasion by the lymphocytes and epitheloid cells.
26. Ans.— A. Argyll Robertson pupil

    Argyll Robertson Pupil (ARP) is slightly small in size and reaction to near reflex is present but light reflex is absent.
27. Ans.— C. Diabetes mellitus
28. Ans.— B. Streptococcus
29. Ans.— E. All of the above
30. Ans.— D. 70
31. Ans.— B. Optic neuritis
32. Ans.— A. Retrobulbar neuritis

    The most common field defect (as in optic neuritis) is central or contracaecal scotoma.
33. Ans.— C. One diopter
34. Ans.— E. None of the above
35. Ans.— D. Sarcoidosis
36. Ans.— C. Lens becomes thinner
37. Ans.— E. Topical medication
38. Ans.— A. The neuroepithelium is normal
39. Ans.— B. Normal pupilary reaction

    Pupil is small, irregular, ectropion or occlusion. Pupillary reaction becomes sluggish or may even be absent due to oedema and hyperemia of iris which hamper its movements.
40. Ans.— A. Neovascularization
41. Ans.— B. Trauma

42. Ans.— D. It requires surgical replacement

43. Ans.— A. Sacroiliac joint

44. Ans.— D. Inferio-nasally

45. Ans.— A. Pilocarpine

46. Ans.— A. Ring synechiae

In Annular posterior synechiae, the aqueous collects behind the iris and pushes it anteriorly leading to iris bombe formation.

47. Ans.— B. Steroids should be avoided

48. Ans.— B. X-ray sacroiliac joint

49. Ans.— D. Aqueous flare

50. Ans.— A. Constricted

51. Ans.— C. The terms iridocyclitis and anterior uveitis are synonymous.

52. Ans.— A. Aqueous flare

One should always look for mutton fat KPs.

53. Ans.— A. Pontine haemorrhage

54. Ans.— A. Granulomatous iritis

55. Ans.— E. Vitreous degeneration

56. Ans.— D. All of the above

In elderly bodies, snow-ball like minute white opacities appear in large numbers, in a vitreous of normal consistency, so that when the eye moves, the opacities move the eyeball. These particles consist of soaps and salts of higher fatty acids. There is no visual disturbance.

57. Ans.— A. Dilate

58. Ans.— D. All of the above

59. Ans.— B. Atropine

In iridocyclitis, atropine : (i) gives comfort and rest to the eye by relieving iris sphincter and ciliary muscle spasm; (ii) prevents the formation of synechiae and may break the already formed synechiae; (iii) reduces exudation by decreasing hyperaemia and vascular permeability and (iv) increases the blood supply to anterior uvea by relieving pressure on the anterior ciliary arteries. As a result more antibodies reach the target tissues and more toxins are absorbed.

60. Ans.— D. Use of oxygen therapy in premature

61. Ans.— A. Iris is broken from ciliary body

62. Ans.— A. Corneal ulcer

63. Ans.— B. Hypopigmented iris

64. Ans.— C. Slit lamp with contact lens

65. Ans.— D. Adie pupil

66. Ans.— D. Opiates

67. Ans.— C. Pseudo. pyocyanea

68. Ans.— D. High myopia

69. Ans.— D. Trauma

70. Ans.— B. Anxiety

71. Ans.— C. Iritis

72. Ans.— C. Miosis

Pupil may be narrow, irregular, ectropion pupillae or occlusio pupil.

73. Ans.— D. High myopia

74. Ans.— A. Pauciarticular juvenile rheumatoid arthritis (JRA).

75. Ans.— B. CRAO

Neovascularization of iris (rubeosis iridis) develops in some eyes with chronic iridocyclitis. Sickle cell retinopathy and Eales' disease are other causes.

76. Ans.— A. Pars planitis

77. Ans.— A. Bowman's membrane

78. Ans.— D. Still's disease

79. Ans.— D. Herpetic uveitis

80. Ans.— C. Base (Root)

81. Ans.— E. All of the above

82. Ans.— A. Acute anterior uveitis

83. Ans.— A. Granulomatous uveitis

84. Ans.— A. More common in females

85. Ans.— A. Progressive atrophy of iris stroma

86. Ans.— D. Myopia

* Uveal effusion is associated with nanophthalmos and not myopia in which there is larger eyeball

87. Ans.— A. Continuation of pigment epithelium

It is anterior continuation of pigment epithelium. Non-pigment in inner layer which forms aquous.

7

IMPORTANT TEXT OF LENS

ANATOMY OF THE LENS

The lens is a biconvex transparent structure, made of lens fibres, which are modified epithelial cells. It is enclosed in an elastic capsule. The anterior surface of the lens is less convex than the posterior and the lens is kept in position, by the suspensory ligament or zonule, which extending from the ciliary process, is attached to the equator of the lens all around. Underneath the anterior capsule, there is a layer of cubical epithelium. The cells near the equator give rise to new lens fibres.

The lens matter consists of a superficial part—the cortex and deeper part the nucleus.

CATARACT

Definition—It means opacity of the lens. Thelens, being an avascular structure, cannot develop an inflammatory disease. The **commonest** disease is a degenerative process leading to opacity of lens fibres, known as cataract.

Classification of cataract

A. **Congenital and Developmental**
This type includes :
1. Blue-dot cataract
2. Coronary cataract
3. Capsular or polar cataract—anterior and posterior
4. Sutural cataract
5. Coralliform cataract
6. Floriform cataract
7. Central cataract
8. Lamellar or zonular cataract
9. Total cataract
   a. Soft
   b. Membranous

B. **Acquired Cataract**
This type includes :
1. Senile cataract
   a) Cortical or cuneiform
   b) Nuclear
   c) Posterior cortical or cupuliform
2. Traumatic cataract
   a. Mechanical trauma—Concussion, convusion or penetrating injury of the eye ball.
   b. Chemical trauma—Due to systemic absorption of chemicals like naphthalene, lactose, galactose, or thallium
   c. Radiational trauma—By infra-red rays, ultra-violet rays, deep X-rays or radiations from radium.
   d. Electric cataract—Due to passage of electric current through the body.
3. Endocrine cataract—As in diabetes mellitus, hypoparathyroidism, and cretinism.
4. Cataract due to systemic disease—As in Mongolian idiocy, myotonic dystrophy and generalized dermatitis.
5. Complicated cataract.

OIL DROPLET IN LENS

1. Anterior displacement of lens
2. Galactosemia-transferase deficiency (von Reuss syndrome)
3. Lenticonus

LENTICONUS (Conical, lens surface protuberance) AND LENTIGLOBUS (Globular lens surface Protuberance)

1. Anterior—Rare and usually bilateral
   A. Alport syndrome (hereditary nephritis)
   B. Spina bifida
   C. Wardenburg syndrome (embryonic fixation syndrome).
2. Posterior—More common and often unilateral.
   A. May be associated with persistent hyperplastic primary vitreous.
   B. May be associated with remnants of hyloid artery.
   C. Lowe syndrome (oculocerebrorenal syndrome).
   D. Trauma

LENS ABSORPTION

1. Congenital rubella syndrome (German measles)
2. Hallerman-Streiff syndrome (dyscephalic mandibulo-oculo facial syndrome)
3. Surgical trauma as discission
4. Trauma, blunt or penetrating

MICROPHAKIA OR SPHEROPHAKIA (Small Lens or Highly Spherical Lens)

1. Achard syndrome (Marfan syndrome with dysostosis mandibulofacilis)
2. Alport syndrome (hereditary nephritis)
3. Familial anomaly
4. Homocystinuria syndrome
5. Hyperlysinemia
6. Lenticular myopia as recessive inheritance trait
7. Little syndrome (hereditary osteo-orcychodysplasia)
8. Lowe syndrome (renal ricketts)
9. Marchesani syndrome (brachymorphy with spherophakia)
10. Marfan syndrome (dolichostenomelia-arachnodactyly hyperchondroplasia dystrophica mesodermalis congenita)
11. Reticular dystrophy of the retinal pigment epithelium
12. Rubella syndrome (Gregg syndrome)
13. Waardenburg syndrome (Embryonic fixation syndrome)

DISLOCATED LENS

1. Achard syndrome (Marfan with dysostosis)
2. Apert syndrome (Sphenoacrocraniosyndactyly)
3. Ascariasis

4. Associated ocular findings
   A. Aniridia
   B. Coloboma of iris and choroid
   C. Congenital glaucoma
   D. High myopia
   E. Megalocornea
   F. Microcornea
5. Autosomal recessive or dominant abnormality without other defects, except usually ectopic pupils.
6. Capsular exfoliation syndrome.
7. Cryptophthalmia syndrome (eyptophthalmos-syndactyly syndrome).
8. Dwarfism, genetic type
9. Ehlers-Danlos syndrome (cutis hyperelastica).
10. Gillum-Anderson syndrome (blepharoptosis, myopia, ectopia lentis).
11. Gronblad-Strandberg syndrome (pseudoxanthoma elasticum).
12. Hereditary ectodermal dysplasia syndrome.
13. Homocystinuria—usually downward displacement of lens.
14. Hyperlysinemia
15. Mandibulofacial dysostosis (Franceschetti syndrome).
16. Marchesani syndrome (brachymorphy with spherophakia).
17. Marfan syndrome (dolichostenomelia-arachnodactyly-hyperchondroplasia dystrophia mesodermalis congenita)—usually superior displacement of lens.
18. Molybdenum cofactor deficiency (combined deficiency of sulfite oxidase and xanthine dehydrogenase).
19. Oculodental syndrome (Peter's syndrome)
20. Recession of anterior syndrome
21. Retinal disinsertion syndrome
22. Rieger syndrome (dysgenesis mesostromalis)
23. Spherophakia
24. Spontaneous (degenerative)
25. Sulfite oxidase deficiency
26. Surgical accidents (iatrogenic)
27. Syphilis (lues)
28. Trauma as in Frenkel syndrome (ocular contusion syndrome) bee sting, and following YAG laser.
29. Treacher-Collins syndrome (mandibulofacial dysostosis).
30. Wildervanck syndrome (cervico-oculoacoustic syndrome).

APHAKIA

Definition

Aphakia is the condition in which the crystalline lens is absent from its normal position.

How aphakia can be produced

1. By operative measures like discission, extra-capsular or intra-capsular extraction of lens.
2. By trauma—Usually contusional injury, when the lens may be dislocated in the vitreous.
3. By couching—When the lens is forcibly dislocated into the vitreous, by a needle introduced through the limbus.
4. As a developmental anomaly—Congenital absence of the lens.

Symptoms of aphakia

There is a marked deemness of vision, both for the distance and for the near, due to development of acquired hypermetropia and due to complete loss of accommodation.

Clinical signs of aphakia

1. Deep anterior chamber
2. Tremulousness of iris known as *iridodonesis.*
3. Jet-black pupil, provided there is no after-cataract.
4. Absence of 3rd and 4th Purkinje's images.
5. Linear scar mark at the upper-half of the limbus, in case where extraction of the lens is the cause of aphakia.

Changes occurring in an aphakic eye

1. Acquired high hypermetropia —The total dioptric power of a normal eye is about **+58 to +60 D,** of which cornea contributes **+42 to +43 D** and the lens in situ contributes **+15 to +18 D.** Thus when the lens is removed, the dioptric power of the eye decreases and so the eye becomes hypermetropic
2. Acquired astigmatism in cases where aphakia is due to extraction of the lens—The astigmatism is against the rule, i.e. the vertical curvature of the cornea is flatter than the horizontal. This is caused by the contraction of the limbal scar.
3. Complete loss of accommodation, as there is no lens.
4. The anterior and the posterior focal lengths of the eyeball increase than normal. Thus the anterior and the posterior focal lengths of the aphakic eye become **23.3 mm** and **31 mm** as compared to **15 mm** and **24 mm** in the normal eye approximately from the cornea.
5. The retinal image of an object in an aphakic eye, even after correction with glasses, becomes bigger by **25-30 percent** than that in the normal eye.

Treatment of aphakia

Aphakia is treated by prescribing spectacle lenses :

(a) The lens to be used for distant vision, provided the eye was emmetropic before operation, is **+10.0 Dsp with +2.0 or +3.0 Dcyl axis 180°**. The +10 dioptre spherical lens is for the correction of the acquired hypermetropia and the +2.0 or +3.0 dioptre cylinder with axis 180°, is for correction of the acquired astigmatism.

(b) The lens for near vision + **13.0 Dsp with + 2.0 or + 3.0 Dcyl axis 180°**. The higher spherical lens is necessary for substituting accommodation. The astigmatic correction remains the same as for the distance.

(c) In aphakia not due to extraction of lens, e.g. due to discission operation, due to couching or due to traumatic dislocation of the lens, the astigmatic correction is not necessary. So + 10.0 Dsp for distance and +13.0 Dst for near work serve the purpose.

(d) To restore binocular vision, when one eye is normal and the other eye is aphakic, either contact lens for the aphakic eye, which reduces the image size difference between the two eyes to about 12 per cent or intro-ocular acrylic lens, introduced into the anterior chamber, may be used, which reduces the image size difference to 2-3 per cent.

N.B Although, the dioptric power of the lens in situ is about + **18 D** a lens of dioptric power + 10 D serves the purpose to correct aphakia as this lens is placed outside the eye.

MCQ's OF LENS

What is important in Lens

Anatomy, Cataract (Congenital, Senile, Complicated), Aphakia, Dislocation

1. **Lenticular rosette formation is usually associated with : TN 1988; Kerala 1989; PGI 2000**
   A. Concussion (Traumatic) cataract
   B. Complicated cataract
   C. Diabetic cataract
   D. Congenital cataract
2. **Spherophalera cataract is seen in : Delhi 1996, 99**
   A. Down's syndrome B. Alport's syndrome
   C. Marfan's syndrome D. Niemann Pick's disease
3. **Cataract is seen in all except : AIIMS 1995, 97**
   A. Galactosemia
   B. Hypoparathyroidism
   C. Rh. arthritis
   D. Glucocorticoid administration
4. **A 3 years old child presents with complete cortical opacity. Treatment best used is : MAHE 1998**
   A. Await spontaneous resolution
   B. Correct refractive error
   C. Aspiration
   D. Lensectomy
5. **Ring of Sommerring is type of : Delhi 1983, 87, 96**
   A. After-cataract B. Congenital cataract
   C. Complicated cataract D. None of the above
6. **The earliest change in a developing senile cortical cataract is : AIIMS 1986, 91**
   A. Intumescence
   B. Development of lens striae
   C. Lamellar separation
   D. Incipient stage
   E. None of the above
7. **Treatment with steroid causes ——— cataract. AI 1996, WB 1996**
   A. Zonular B. Post. subcapsular
   C. Lamellar D. Coralliform
8. **The thinnest part of lens capsule is : BHU 1996**
   A. Anterior part
   B. Posterior part
   C. Peripheral part
   D. All have equal thickness
9. **Metabolism of lens is from : JIPMER 1997**
   A. Coricycle B. Glycolysis
   C. EMP shunt D. Atmospheric air
10. **Which of the following statement is false regarding soft contact lenses : Rajasthan 1994**
    A. Made up of HEMA.
    B. Suitable for long term wear due to permeability to O2.
    C. Prolonged adaptation period not required.
    D. More durable & less serious complication than hard lenses.
11. **During lens extractiôn vitreous loss lead to following except : AIIMS 1997**
    A. Asteroid hyalitis B. Updrawn pupil
    C. Retinal detachment D. Visual defect
12. **After Aphakia, refraction is maximally achieved as : Delhi 1989**
    A. 6/6 B. 6/12
    C. 6/18 D. 6.80
13. **Commonest complication of posterior intraocular implant is : Delhi 1988, 90**
    A. After cataract
    B. Retinal compliance
    C. Hyphaema syndrome
    D. Dislocation
14. **Cataract is associated with : PGI 1988, 89**
    A. Pseudo muscular hypertrophy
    B. Myotonia congenita
    C. Myotonic dystrophy
    D. SLE

Ans.	1. A	2. B	3. C	4. D	5. A	6. C	7. B	8. B	9. B	10. D
	11. A	12. A	13. D	14. C						

15. **Atopic cataract is that which follows :** **Karnataka 1998**
A. Esposure to syphilis
B. Injury
C. Poisoning
D. Skin diseases like Eczema

16. **The commonest type of cataract in children is :** **PGI 1984, 85**
A. Snow flake cataract B. Lamellar cataract
C. Morgagnian cataract D. Sunflower cataract

17. **Which of the following is not correctable in Aphakia :** **UP 1998**
A. Loss of accommodation
B. Retinal enlargement of image
C. Reduced vision
D. Pin cushion effect

18. **Treatment of choice in Aphakia is :** **AIIMS 1992**
A. Spectacles B. Contact lens
C. Anterior chamber IOL D. Posterior chamber IOL

19. **Following are associated with Zonular cataract except :** **PGI 1993**
A. IUGR B. Rickets
C. Dental abnormality D. Diabetes

20. **Len's dislocation seen in which syndrome :** **AI 1989, 93**
A. Down's B. Edward's
C. Marfan's D. Turner

21. **Anterior polar cataract develops after :** **AI 1993**
A. Penetrating injury of cornea
B. DM
C. Irradiation
D. Chalc

22. **After cataract operation lens are prescribed after :** **AI 1993**
A. 2 weeks B. 4 weeks
C. 6 weeks D. 12 weeks

23. **Commonest congenital cataract is :** **Delhi 1993**
A. Nuclear B. Zonular
C. Capular D. Coralliform

24. **Commonest indication of intraocular implant is :** **Delhi 1993**
A. Diabetic cataract B. Unilateral cataract
C. Complicated cataract D. Dislocation of lens

25. **Lens has a respiratory quotient of :** **AIIMS 1983**
A. 1 B. 0.6
C. 0.7 D. 0.9

26. **All are true about a cataractous subluxated lens except :** **Delhi 1984**
A. Should be extracted with a wire vectis or cryoprobe.
B. May result from chronic uveitis.
C. If untreated, may cause bullous keratopathy.
D. Should be treated conservatively with typical miotics.

27. **Synchisis scintillans is :** **Rohtak 1986**
A. Associated with solid vitreous
B. Associated with fluidity of vitreous
C. Seen in migraine
D. Related to scintillating scotoma
E. None of the above

28. **Cataract bruncscens result to deposition of :** **AIIMS 1986**
A. Melanin B. Copper
C. Iron D. Silver
E. Gold

29. **During the intracapsular extraction of a lens, undue traction on the capsule may cause all, except :** **AIIMS 1986**
A. Intraocular haemorrhage
B. Separation of vitreous from the retina
C. Holes in the serrata
D. Tears in the anterior hyaloid of the vitreous

30. **After the completion of cataract extraction all of the following points of wound hygiene are important, except :** **AIIMS 1985**
A. The iris must be reposited carefully.
B. Air should be injected behind the iris.
C. The sutures are carefully tied and cut.
D. The conjunctiva and capsular remnants must be removed from the wound.

31. **All of the following are true about suction in aspiration of congenital cataract, except :** **PGI 1986**
A. The iris must be avoided
B. The needle opening should be forward
C. The needle opening should be posterior
D. Suction and injection should be repeated

32. **Cataract is seen in all of the following except :** **Delhi 1994**
A. Renal transplant B. Thyrotoxicosis
C. Irradiation D. Scleroderma

33. **Power of eye is :** **AI 1997**
A. + 52 D B. + 54 D
C. + 56 D D. + 58 D

34. **Hard contact lenses should be avoided in :** **MAHE 1992**
A. Elderly patients
B. Emmetropic patients
C. Patients with unilateral aphakia
D. Patients who require regular eye drops

Ans.									
15. D	16. B	17. A	18. D	19. D	20. C	21. A	22. C	23. B	24. B
25. A	26. D	27. B	28. A	29. A	30. B	31. C	32. B	33. C	34. A

35. In congenital cataract, multiple needling may cause all of the following except : AIIMS 1982
A. Optic neuritis
B. Late retinal detachment
C. Glaucoma
D. Vitreous contact with corneal endothelium

36. Which of the following statement about intra-ocular lens implants is false: MAHE 1992
A. The material used (polymethylmethacrylate) is biologically inert.
B. They usually have a dioptric strength of 19-21 dioptres.
C. They are more often positioned behind the iris.
D. They are sewn into the ciliary body.

37. Which of the following can be a persistent problem in contact lens wearers : MAHE 1996
A. Angular conjunctivitis
B. Conical cornea
C. Follicular conjunctivitis
D. Subconjunctival haemorrhages

38. Senile nuclear sclerosis may result in which type of cataract : DNB 1989
A. Blue dot B. Black
C. Oil drop D. Snow flakes

39. Rediation mainly causes cataract of ——— type. PGI 1993, 94
A. Anterior subcapsular B. Posterior subcapsular
C. Nuclear D. Polar

40. Features of a subluxated lens include all of the following, except : DNB 1990
A. Unipolar diplopia
B. Hypermetropia
C. Irregular anterior chamber
D. Iridodonesis
E. Lens margin may be seen in the pupil

41. Power of intraocular lens used in emmetopic person is : Delhi 1996, 97
A. + 18 D B. + 19.5 D
C. + 20.5 D D. 21. 5 D

42. In cataract important etiological factor is : Delhi 1996
A. Smoking B. Hypertension
C. Trauma D. Hyperparathyroidism

43. The etiology of complicated cataract include all, except : AP 1987
A. Disciform keratitis B. Iridocyclitis
C. Retinitis pigmentosa D. Retinal detachment

44. Cataract associated with convulsions is seen with all except : AIIMS 1994
A. Galactosemia
B. Toxoplasmosis
C. Birth asphyxia and prematurity
D. Tay sach's disease

45. Lens derives its nourishments from : AIIMS 1980
A. Air
B. Perilimbal capillaries
C. Vitreous humour
D. Aqueous humour

46. Day blindness is a feature of : AIIMS 1980
A. Cortical cataract B. Cupuliform cataract
C. Blue dot cataract D. Coralliform cataract
E. None of the above

47. Cataract is produced in experimental animals by avoiding : Karnataka 1996
A. Glycine B. Cystine
C. Threonine D. Tryptophan

48. Least common complication of congenital cataract surgery is : AIIMS 1981
A. Pupillary occlusion B. Glaucoma
C. Phthisis bulbi D. Pupillary displacement
E. Retinal detachment

49. "Sun flower" cataract is characteristic of : AI 1988
A. Argyrosis B. Siderosis
C. Chalcosis D. None of the above

50. Lens striae appear at first in : AIIMS 1982
A. Upper nasal quadrant
B. Lower nasal quadrant
C. Upper temporal quadrant
D. Lower temporal quadrant
E. None of the above

51. The ageing lens may show all of the following, except : Rohtak 1988
A. Increase in insoluble albuminoid
B. Decrease in ascorbic acid
C. Increase in bulk
D. Increase in total protein content
E. Increase in soluble proteins

52. In which of the following diseases, sorbitol accumulates in the lens of the eye : TNPSC 1997
A. Wilson's disease B. von Gierke's disease
C. Galactosemia D. Diabetes mellitus

53. Hard contact lenses are made-up of : AIIMS 1985
A. HEMA B. PMMA
C. Silicon D. Glass

Ans.									
35. A	36. A	37. C	38. B	39. B	40. B	41. A	42. C	43. A	44. D
45. D	46. B	47. D	48. C	49. C	50. B	51. E	52. D	53. B	

54. **'Oil drop' cataract is seen in : AIIMS 1985, 87**
A. Diabetes mellitus B. Injuries
C. Galactosemia D. Eye infections

55. **A typical diabetic cataract has the following characteristic morphology : AIIMS 1985**
A. Sunflower B. Snow flake
C. Irregular D. Rusty

56. **Anterior polar cataract is commonly seen with : AIIMS 1988**
A. Perforation of cornea
B. Trachoma
C. Choriolenticular cataract
D. Irradiation

57. **Lens develops from : AIIMS 1988**
A. Neuroectoderm B. Surface ectoderm
C. Mesoderm D. Endoderm

58. **Premature cataract is seen with : PGI 1988**
A. Turner's syndrome B. Klinefelter syndrome
C. Frohlich's syndrome D. Reiter's syndrome

59. **Best management of a congenital cataract is : UP 1998**
A. Within 24 hours B. At one month
C. After 6 months D. At One year

60. **Contact lens associated with all except : DNB 1994**
A. ↓ Oxygen B. ↓ Glucose uptake
C. Corneal oedema D. ↑ Endothelial cell loss
E. ↓ Corneal sensitivity

61. **In phakoemulsification surgery, following sutures are of choice : Delhi 1995**
A. No sutures B. Multiple interrupted
C. Continuous sutures D. Non-absorbable sutures

62. **The commonest type of cataract in adults is : PGI 1986**
A. Nuclear cataract B. Cortical cataract
C. Morgangian cataract D. None of the above

63. **Most important measure to prevent infection following cataract surgery is : Delhi 1997**
A. Subconjuctival injection of 20 mg gentamicin.
B. Preoperative administration of antibiotic eye drops.
C. Pre-operative intraocular administration of antibiotics.
D. Systemic antibiotics post-operatively.

64. **Contact lens is best used in : AIIMS 1984, 89**
A. High myopia
B. Aphakia
C. Irregular astigmatism
D. High astigmatism

65. **In which of the following type of intraocular lens implant is extracapsular lens extraction used : AIIMS 1985, 89**
A. Iris support B. Anterior synechia
C. Posterior chamber D. Angle support

66. **Thickness of lens in an adult is : AMU 1986**
A. 2.25 mm B. 3.15 mm
C. 4.25 mm D. 6.25 mm

67. **Intraocular lens is contraindicated in : DNB 1989**
A. Young diabetics
B. One eyed
C. Overt corneal dystrophy
D. All of the above

68. **Mental retardation associated with a fair complexion and aphakia to be due to which of the following : DNB 1989**
A. Phenylketonuria B. Galactosemia
C. Homocystinuria D. Albinims
E. All of the above

69. **Good vision during night is present in : Delhi 1985, 87**
A. Central cataract
B. Complicated cataract
C. Rosette shaped cataract
D. Snow flake cataract

70. **On removing lens, the image size is increased by : Rajasthan 1990**
A. 10% B. 20%
C. 30% D. 50%

71. **Cylindrical lenses are used in : PGI 1982**
A. Astigmatism B. Myopia
C. Hypermetropia D. Presbyopia

72. **Vision is diminished in day light in which type of cataract : PGI 1985, 88**
A. Peripheral B. Central
C. Hypermature D. Concussion

73. **Nuclear cataract is associated with the following type of refractive error : AP 1994**
A. Myopia B. Hypermetropia
C. Presbyopia D. Astigmatism

74. **A 50 year old person with features of coloured halos was examined for Finchams test which revealed that halos break-up and then rejoin. Diagnosis is : AIIMS 1993**
A. Senile immature cataract
B. Open angle glaucoma
C. Ac. congestive glaucoma
D. Mucopurulent conjunctivitis

Ans.									
54. C	55. B	56. A	57. B	58. C	59. B	60. B	61. B	62. B	63. A
64. A	65. C	66. C	67. D	68. C	69. A	70. C	71. A	72. D	73. A
74. A									

75. Exact site where intraocular lens is commonly fitted : Delhi 1994

A. Capsular ligament B. Endosulcus
C. Ciliary supported D. Capsular bag

76. Immature cataract can be diagnosed by : TN 1999

A. Retinoscopy
B. Direct ophthalmoscopy
C. Distant direct opthalmoscopy
D. Indirect ophthalmoscopy

77. Double vision is seen in ——— cataract: AP 1999

A. Nuclear B. Cortical
C. Punctate D. Complete

78. Phacoemulsification usually takes: Delhi 2000

A. 1-3 min B. 3-5 min
C. 10-15 min D. 15-20 min

79. Common complications of IOL lens are except : PGI 2000

A. Corneal dystrophy B. Glaucoma
C. Aniseiconia D. Macular edema

80. Christmas tree cataract is found in : UP 1999; PGI 1999

A. Wilson's disease B. Diabetic
C. Traumatic D. Myotonic dystrophy

81. Earliest visual rehabilitation occurs with : UP 2000

A. Phacoemulsification B. ICCE+IOL
C. ECCE+IOL D. ICCE alone or laser

82. 'Second sight' is seen in : MAHE 2000

A. Cortical cataract B. Morgagnian cataract
C. Nuclear cataract D. Zonular cataract

83. Cataract can be caused by prolonged ingestion of which drug : Delhi 2001

A. Phenothiazines B. Methotrexate
C. Ethambutol D. Chloroquine

84. When aphakic eye is corrected with IOL, what all happens: Kerala 2001

A. Distant vision obtained
B. Both distant and near vision good
C. Distant vision with field of vision
D. Distant with acquity

85. In a patient with cataract, capsulotomy with removal of lens nucleus followed by aspiration of cortical content is known as : SGPGI 2002

A. Intracapsular cataract extraction
B. Extracapsular cataract extraction
C. Discission
D. Lensectomy

86. Power of intraocular lens is determined by : Rajasthan 2001

A. A mode USG B. B mode USG
C. C mode USG D. D mode USG

87. Which morphological type of cataract is more visually handicapping : AIIMS 2002

A. Cortical B. Nuclear
C. Posterior subcapsular D. Zonular

88. The standard sutureless cataract surgery done with phaco-emulsification and foldable IOL has an incision of : AIIMS 2002

A. 1 mm - 1.5 mm B. 2 mm - 2.5 mm
C. 3 mm - 3.5 mm D. 3.5 mm - 4.5 mm

89. A child has got a congenital cataract involving the visual axis which was detected by the parents right at birth. This child should be operated : AI 2003

A. Immediately
B. At 2 months of age.
C. At 1 yr of age when the globle becomes normal sized.
D. After 4 yrs of age when the entire ocular and orbital grow.

90. Polychromatic lustre is seen in : AI 2004

A. Complicated cataract B. Diabetes mellitus
C. Post radiation cataract D. Congenital cataract

91. A two weeks old child presents with unilateral cataract, Which of the following statement represents the best management advice: AI 2004

A. The best age to operate him to get the best visual results is four weeks.
B. The best age to operate him to get the best visual results is four months.
C. The best age to operate him to get the best visual results is four years.
D. The eye is already lost, only cosmetic correction is required.

92. Contact lens wear is proven to have deleterious effects on the corneal physiology. Which of the following statements is incorrect in connection with contact lens wear: AI 2005

A. The level of glucose availability in the corneal epithelium is reduced.
B. There is a reduction in hemidesmosome density.
C. There is increased production of CO2 in the epithelium.
D. There is a reduction in glucose utilization by corneal epithelium.

Ans.									
75 D	76. C	77. B	78. B	79. C	80. D	81. A	82. C	83. A	84. B
85. B	86. B	87. A	88. B	89. A	90. A	91. A	92. A		

93. Congenital cataract with involvement of visual axis, What to do : DNB 2011

A. Immediated operate
B. Wait & watch
C. Mydriatics
D. Operate in adulthood

94. The appearence of cortical cataract show up as spokes of a wheel diagnosis is : AI 2012

A. Lamellar cataract
B. Complicated cataract
C. None of the above
D. All of the above

95. Irregular branching hyphae infection in contact lens users is : AI 2012

A. Acanthoemeba
B. Angular conjuncitivitis
C. Fungal ulcers
D. Trachoma

96. A 70 years old boy after successful phacoemulsification and IOL placement. After few days pain and vision deteriortes petals of flowers pattern and FFA and with aquous flare and posteriorsynechial cause is : AI 2012

A. Cystoid macular edema
B. Central serous retinopathy
C. Postopertaive panopthalmitis
D. Endopthalmitis

97. A 70-year old male after cataract surgery complained of decreased vision and flower petal appearance on FFA is due to : AI 2012

A. Central serous retinopathy
B. Cystoid macular oedema
C. Endophthalmitis
D. Sympathetic ophthalmia

Ans. 93. A 94. A 95. A 96. C 97. B

EXPLANATIONS OF LENS

1. Ans. — A. Concussion (Traumatic) cataract

   Early rosette cataract (punctate) is the most typical form of concussion cataract. In develops in posterior cortex. Late rosette cataract develops in posterior cortex 1-2 years after injury.

2. Ans. — B. Alport's syndrome
3. Ans. — C. Rh. arthritis
4. Ans. — D. Lensectomy
5. Ans. — A. After-cataract
6. Ans. — C. Lamellar separation
7. Ans. — B. Post. subcapsular
8. Ans. — B. Posterior part
9. Ans. — B. Glycolysis
10. Ans. — D. More durable & less serious complication than hard lenses
11. Ans. — A. Asteroid hyalitis
12. Ans. — A. 6/6
13. Ans. — D. Dislocation
14. Ans. — C. Myotonic dystrophy

    In myotonic dystrophy, a sharply limited zone of cortex underneath the capsule both anteriorly and posteriorly, with tiny iridescent spots. The cataract may remain stationary, if it progresses, the operative prognosis is good.

15. Ans. — D. Skin diseases like Eczema
16. Ans. — B. Lamellar cataract
17. Ans. — A. Loss of accommodation
18. Ans. — D. Posterior chamber IOL

    Hard lenses are made up of PMMA while soft lenses from HEMA.

19. Ans. — D. Diabetes
20. Ans. — C. Marfan's

    Ectopia lentis is usually upwards displacement and bilateral. Other features are arachnodactyly of hands and feet, dolichocephalic skull, flat foot, congenital anomalies of heart.

21. Ans. — A. Penetrating injury of cornea
22. Ans. — C. 6 weeks
23. Ans. — B. Zonular
24. Ans. — B. Unilateral cataract
25. Ans. — A. 1
26. Ans. — D. Should be treated conservatively with typical miotics.
27. Ans. — B. Associated with fluidity of vitreous
28. Ans. — A. Melanin

    Cataracta brunescens is brown in colour. Cataracta -nigra is black and cataracta rubra is red in colour.

29. Ans. — A. Intraocular haemorrhage
30. Ans. — B. Air should be injected behind the iris.
31. Ans. — C. The needle opening should be posterior.
32. Ans. — B. Thyrotoxicosis
33. Ans. — C. + 56 D

    Diopteric power of eye is +58 to +60 D of which cornea contributes + 42 to +43 and lens in situ +15 to -18D.

34. Ans. — A. Elderly patients
35. Ans. — A. Optic neuritis
36. Ans. — A. The material used (polymethylmethacrylate) is biologically inert.
37. Ans. — C. Follicular conjunctivitis
38. Ans. — B. Black
39. Ans. — B. Posterior subcapsular

    Exposure to almost all types of radiant energy is known to produce cataract by causing damage to lens epithelium. Types are infrared (heat) cataract causing discoid posterior subcapsular cataract (Glass blower's or glass worker's cataract). Irradiation cataract occurs on exposure to X-ray, Gamma rays or neutrons (with latent period from 6 months to a few years) and ultraviolet radiation cataract.

40. Ans. — B. Hypermetropia

41. Ans.— A. + 18 D

42. Ans.— C. Trauma

43. Ans.— A. Disciform keratitis

44. Ans.— D. Tay sach's disease

In galactosemia, oil droplet central lens opacities or cataract are seen.

45. Ans.— D. Aqueous humour

46. Ans.— B. Cupuliform cataract

47. Ans.— D. Tryptophan

48. Ans.— C. Phthisis bulbi

49. Ans.— C. Chalcosis

In injuries, there is Rosette-shaped cataract whereas in diabetes, it is Snow-flake type and in Galactosemia, Oil drop type.

50. Ans.— B. Lower nasal quadrant

51. Ans.— E. Increase in soluble proteins

52. Ans.— D. Diabetes mellitus

53. Ans.— B. PMMA

54. Ans.— C. Galactosemia

55. Ans.— B. Snow flake

56. Ans.— A. Perforation of cornea

57. Ans.— B. Surface ectoderm

58. Ans.— C. Frohlich's syndrome

59. Ans.— B. At one month

60. Ans.— B. ↓ Glucose uptake

61. Ans.— B. Multiple interrupted

62. Ans.— B. Cortical cataract

63. Ans.— A. Subconjuctival injection of 20 mg gentamicin

64. Ans.— A. High myopia

65. Ans.— C. Posterior chamber

66. Ans.— C. 4.25 mm

The diameter of lens is 9-10 mm and thickness varies with age from 3.5 mm (at birth) to 5 mm (at extreme of age). Its weight varies from 135 mg (0-9 years) to 255 mg (40-80 years of age). Radius of curvature in anterior surface is 10 mm and of posterior surface is 6 mm. Its refractive index is 1.39 and total power is 15-16 D. The accomodative power of lens varies with age, being 14-16D (at birth), 7-8D (at 25 years of age) and 1-2 D (at 50 years of age).

67. Ans.— D. All of the above

68. Ans.— C. Homocystinuria

69. Ans.— A. Central cataract

70. Ans.— C. 30%

71. Ans.— A. Astigmatism

72. Ans.— D. Concussion

73. Ans.— A. Myopia

74. Ans.— A. Senile immature cataract

75. Ans.— D. Capsular bag

76. Ans.— C. Distant direct opthalmoscopy

77. Ans.— B. Cortical

78. Ans.— B. 3-5 min

Phacoemulsification is presently the most pupular method of extracapsular cataract extraction.

79. Ans.— C. Aniseikonia

80. Ans.— D. Myotonic dystrophy

81. Ans.— A. Phacoemulsification

82. Ans.— C. Nuclear cataract

83. Ans.— A. Phenothiazines

84. Ans.— B. Both distant and near vision good

85. Ans.— B. Extracapsular cataract extraction

86. Ans.— B. B mode USG

87. Ans.— A. Cortical

88. Ans.— B. 2 mm - 2.5 mm

89. Ans.— A. Immediately

Complete bilateral cataracts should be removed as early as possible (within few weeks of birth) to prevent stimulus deprivation amblyopia.

90. Ans.— A. Complicated cataract :

Complicated cataract

- It is secondary to the inflammatory or degenerative diseases of eye such as iridocyclitis, choroiditis, high myopia, retinal detachment and primary pig-mentary degeneration of retina.
- Characterised by ill-defined opacification of posterior cortical area having "bread-crumb" appearance.
- The slit-lamp examination exhibit a characteristic rainbow display of colour called polychromatic lustre (a diagnostic sign).

Cataracts	*Causes*
Snow flake/snow storm cataract	Diabetes
Sun flower cataract	Wilson's disease
Oil droplet cataract	Galactosaemia
Glass blower's cataract	Infra-red (heat)
Atopic cataract	Atopic dermatitis
Rosette cataract	Concussion injury of lens
Christmas tree cataract	Dystrophica myotunica

91. Ans. — A. The best age to operate him to get the best visual results is four weeks.

Treatment of Congenital cataract :

- Complete unilateral cataract should be preferably removed within a few weeks of birth (as early as possible within the first 6 weeks of birth).
- Complete bilateral congenital cataract should also be removed as early as possible (within few weeks of birth) to prevent stimulus deprivation amblyopia.

92. Ans. — A. The level of glucose availability in the corneal epithelium is reduced.

- Facts about contact lens related disorders.

93. Ans. — A. Immediated operate

Repeat Question.

94. Ans. — A. Lamellar cataract

Lamellar cataract is a form where the opacity only affects some of the layers of the eye lens i.e. the layers outside the nucleus. The spokes of wheel opacity gives rider appearance.

95. Ans. — A. Acanthoemeba

Acanthamoeba survives in space between contact lens and eye. Contact lenses should be removed when swimming or surfing. There is keratitis with severe pain, corneal perineuritis and ring ulcer. Sheep blood agar plate and PCR are used for diagnosis. Treatment is PHMB (Propamidine isethionate) and chlorhexadine keratoplasty may be required.

96. Ans. — C. Postoperative panopthalmitis

It is a postoperative complication.

97. Ans. — B. Cystoid macular oedema

On fundus fluorescence angiography, flower petals appearance is seen in post. cataract surgery cystoid macular oedema. Irvine first descrbied it in 1963. Incidence is 20-30%. It is due to accumulation of fluid in outer plexiform layer and inner retinal layers of perifoveal region whether in swollen and degenerating Muller cells or as extracellular cysts.

COMBINED MEDICAL SERVICES EXAMINATION
(Conducted by UPSC)

- It contains original solved papers from **1983 onwards**
- All papers are **Subjectwise & Yearwise** arranged
- Answers are given at the foot and **detailed explanations** are given at the end.
- Detailed **Instructions** about this examination are given
- Important **references** to be read are also given
- Each year's paper is classified into two separate parts arranged subjectwise
- Book is suited for Quick revision before the examination and also to know its pattern
- High chance of repetition in this exam as well as in other UPSC conducted Exams
- Read the papers before undertaking preparation (to know the pattern), then read text and again check your knowledge by doing papers
- Also useful for **Civil Services Examination, Part I** (Medical Sciences) as the question Bank is same
- Also read book on **Civil Services Examination, Part I (Medical Sciences)** (by same author and publishers) as the **Question Bank** of two exams may overlap.
- All suggestions and Contributions are welcome and write to the Editor :
  Dr. M.S. Bhatia, D-1, Naraina Vihar, New Delhi-110028

CBS Publishers & Distributors Pvt. Ltd.
NEW DELHI • BANGALORE • PUNE • CHENNAI • COCHIN

8

IMPORTANT TEXT OF GLAUCOMA

INTRA-OCULAR PRESSURE

Definition of intra-ocular pressure

It is the pressure above the atmospheric pressure, maintained inside the eyeball in normal condition, created by the volume of the solid and liquid contents of the eye and the elasticity of its coats.

Normal intra-ocular pressure

It varies from **16 to 23 mm of Hg**. It is higher than that developed inside any other organ in the body, for example the normal tissue pressure is **2 to 3 mm of Hg.** and the cerebrospinal fluid pressure is about **7 mm or Hg.** in the recumbent position.

Why this high pressure is in the eye?

Compared to other organs, this high pressure inside the eye is necessary for the maintenance of the optical properties of the refracting surfaces. As for example the curvature of the cornea and the smoothness of its surface must be kept constant and also the water content of the corneal stroma has to be maintained at a constant level to keep the refractive index uniform.

Factors responsible for normal intra-ocular pressure

The pressure inside the eyeball is created by :

a) Elasticity of its outer i.e. cornea and sclera

b) The volume of its solid and liquid contents.

i) Elasticity of the outer coats—

The outer wall of the eye does not act as a rigid boxy and there is a definite although very little distensibility of cornea and sclera. This distensibility exerts an important effect upon the mechanism of intra-ocular pressure.

ii) Volume of intra-ocular contents—

(i) Solid and semi-solid structures like the lens, vitreous, uveal tract and retina which by change in volume may lead to alteration in intra-ocular pressure.

(ii) Fluid contents like blood and aqueous humour and a variation in their volume can alter intraocular pressure considerably.

Factors responsible for maintenance of steady level of normal intra-ocular pressure

Although, there are minor physiological variations of intra-ocular pressure as already described, there is a more or less constant steady level of intra-ocular pressure, in spite of the fact that there is a continuous leakage from the eye. The factors which maintain this steady level are follows :

a) Continuous formation of the aqueous humour by secreatary process of the ciliary epithelium and by ultra-filtration from the ciliary capillaries.

b) The normal resistant offered by the drainage channels for the outflow of the fluid of the eye.

c) The pressure in the episcleral veins in which ultimately the aqueous humour is drained.

GLAUCOMA

Definition—It is a condition where the intra-ocular pressure of the eyeball increases more than normal (normal pressure = **16 to 23 mm of Hg**. by Schiotz tonometer **15-16 mm Hg** by Applanation tonometer.

CLASSIFICATION OF GLAUCOMA

(i)	*Congenital* (Infantile glaucoma or Buphthalmos or Hydrophthalmos)	*Acquired*
(ii)	*Primary* (Without any obvious causes)	*Secondary* (When obvious cause is present)
(iii)	*Wide-angle* or Chronic simple glaucoma	*Closed-angle* or Congestive glaucoma

NB : Absolute glaucoma—It is a stage of glaucoma when sense of perception and projection of light is lost. This condition may occur in the final stage of buphthalmos, wide-angle glaucoma closed-angle glaucoma of secondary glaucoma.

DIFFERENTIAL DIAGNOSIS BETWEEN BUPHTHALMOS AND MEGALOCORNEA

Buphthalmos	*Megalocornea*
1. Familial occurrence rare.	1. Familial occurrence common
2. Males to females = 5 : 3	2. Almost entirely in males
3. Unilateral in 35% of cases	3. Bilateral
4. Corneal opacities and ruptures in Descemet's membrane	4. No corneal opacities
5. Visual impairment is marked	5. No visual impairment
6. Intra-ocular tension raised	6. No rise of tension
7. Gross abnormalities at the angle of the anterior chamber	7. No malformation at the angle
8. Cupping of the disc present	8. No cupping of the disc

Treatment—Not *very* satisfactory

1. Miotics are of no value
2. Operative treatment :

(a) Ordinary fistualizing operation, like trephining or iridencleisis may be tried. But there is tendency for the fistula to close and operations may have to be repeated.

(b) Goniotomy—i.e. to cut through the mesodermal tissue at the angle of the anterior chamber, with the point of a especially constructed knife, introduced through the limbus. If successful, the angle opens and tension becomes controlled.

CONDITIONS SIMULATING CONGENITAL GLAUCOMA

1. Anterior corneal staphyloma
2. Birth injury, such as breaks in Descemet membrane
3. Bloch-Sulzberger syndrome (incontinentia pigmenti)
4. Blue sclerotic syndrome (brittle cornea syndrome)
5. Congenital anomalies, such as sclerocornea
6. Congenital corneal dystrophy
7. Congenital idiopathic corneal edema
8. Corneal amyloidosis (Lubarsch-Pick syndrome)
9. Corneal plana

10. Corneal xanthomas
11. Inflammation
    A. Blepharitis, keratoconjunctivitis, and keratitis on a chemical, allergic, bacterial, or viral basis
    B. Fetal iritis or uveitis
    C. Intrauterine gonorrhea keratitis
    D. Chickenpox viruses—intrauterine
    E. Syphilitic interstitial keratitis
12. Intraocular tumor, such as retinoblastoma or diktyoma
13. Keratoconus
14. Keratoectasia
15. Megalocornea
16. Metabolic disorders
    A. Cystinosis or cystine storage disease
    B. Familial lipoidosis
    C. Hurler disease (MPS-1), Morquio-Brailsford disease (MPS-IV), Schete disease (MPS-V), and Maroteaux lamy disease (MPS-VI)
    D. Porphyria
17. Myopia
18. Riley-Day syndrome (congenital familial dysautonomia)
19. Trisomy 13-15 syndrome (Patau syndrome)
20. von Gierke disease (glycogen disease)

ELEVATED INTRAOCULAR PRESSURE WITH NORMAL OPTIC DISC

1. Excessive water intake
2. High scleral rigidity
3. Hypertension
4. Hyperthyroid
5. Marked emotional stress
6. Mechanical factors in checking intraocular pressure
7. Normal variation
8. Preglaucoma
9. Steroid intake (local, systemic)

GLAUCOMA ASSOCIATED WITH DISPLACED LENS

1. Anterior chamber angle deformity
2. Anterior chamber recessed angle
3. Peripheral posterior synechiae
4. Phacolytic
5. Pupillary block
6. Uveitis

GLAUCOMA ASSOCIATED WITH SHALLOW ANTERIOR CHAMBER

1. Acquired immune-deficiency syndrome.
2. Acute hyperglycemia
3. Anterior chamber intraocular lens vaulting.
4. Cystinosis syndrome (Lignac-Fanconi syndrome).
5. Cilochoroidal effusions mechanically obstructing the chamber angle.
6. Complication of scleral buckling retinal detachment surgery.
7. Lens subluxation or intumescence.
8. Ophthalodynia hypertonic copulationis syndrome.
9. Plateau iris syndrome.
10. Post-operative inflammatory pressure elevation in the presence of a narrow but open angle.
11. Pupillary block
12. Suprachoroidal haemorrhage

APHAKIC GLAUCOMA (Glaucoma in Aphakia)

1. Associated with pseudoexfoliation in aphakia.
2. Epithelialization of anterior chamber.
3. Immediate post-operative reaction following intracapsular extraction from traumatic iritis or alpha-chymotrypsin use.
4. Peripheral anterior synechiae from loss of vitreous, prolapse of iris, incarceration of iris or lens capsule in wound, or absent anterior chamber.
5. Primary open-angle glaucoma.
6. Prolonged post-operative inflammation in aphakia in both intracapsular and extracapsular extraction.
7. Pupillary block
8. Vitreous filling the anterior chamber.

MEDICATION THAT MAY CAUSE GLAUCOMA

Medications that may cause glaucoma include adrenal cortex injection, aldosterone, alpha-chymotrypsin, aluminium nicotinate(?), aminotrate phosphate, amitriptyline, amyl nitrite, atropine, belladonna, benzilonium bromide, betamethasone, carbon dioxide, chlorpromazine, cortisone, cyclopentolate, cyproheptadine hydrochloride, demecarium, desoxycorticosterone, dexamethasone, dibenzheptropine, dicyclomine hydrochloride, echothiophate, erythrityl tetranitrate (?), fludrocortisone, fluorometholone, fluprednisolone, glycopyrolate, glyceryltrinitrite, homatropine, hydrocortisone, hydroxyamphetamine, hyoscyamine, imipramine, isoflurophate, isopropamide iodide, isosorbide dinitrate (?), ketamine, mannitol hexanitrate (?), medrysone, mepenzolate, methixenehydrochloride, methylphenidate (?), methylprednisolone, morphine (?), niacinamide (?), nicotinic acid (?), nicotinyl alcohol (?), nitroglycerin, nitrous oxide, nortriptyline, orphenadrine, oxyphencyclimine, oxyphenonium, paramethasone, penta-erythritoltetranitrate (?), penthianate bromide, phenothiazine, phenylephrine, phenylephrine, pilocarpine, pipenzolate bromide, phenothiazine, phenylephrine, pilocarpine, pipenzolate bromide, prednisolone, prednisone, propantheline bromide, scopolamine, sodium chloride, succinylcholine, testosterone (?), tolazoline, triamcinolone, trimipramine, trolnitrate (?), tropicamide; urokinase

CHERRY RED SPOT IN MACULA (RULE OUT MACULAR HAEMORRHAGE)

1. β-Galactoosidase deficiency (mucopolysaccharidoses 9 MPS) VII
2. Cardiac myxomas
3. Cryoglobulinemia
4. Hallevorden-Spartz disease (pigmentary degeneration of globus pallidus)
5. Hollenhorst syndrome (chorioretinal infarction syndrome)
6. Hurler syndrome (MPS I-H)
7. Hypertension (severe)
8. Intralesional chalazion corticosteroid injection
9. Macular retinal hole with surrounding detachment
10. Mucolipidosis-I (lipomucopolysaccharidosis)
11. Myotonic dystrophy syndromy (Curschmann-Steinert syndrome)
12. Occlusion of central retinal artery
13. Quinine toxicity
14. Sphingo-lipidoses
    A. Cherry-red spot myoclonus
    B. Farber syndrome (Farber lipogranulomatosis)
    C. Gangliosidosis (GMI—type 2 (juvenile gangliosidosis)
    D. Gaucher's disease (glucocerebroside storage disease)
    E. Goldberg syndrome
    F. Infantile metachromatic leukodystrophy (van Bogaert-Nijssen disease)
    G. Niemann-Pick disease (essential lipoid histiocytosis)
    H. Sandoff disease (gangliosidosis GM2—type 2)
    I. Tay-Sachs disease (familial amaurotic idiocy)
15. Temporal arteries (Hutchinson—Horton Magrath-Brown syndrome)
16. Traumatic retinal edema (commotio retinae; Berlin edema)
17. Vogt-Spielmeyer cerebral degeneration (Batten-Mayou syndrome).

MCQ's OF GLAUCOMA

What is important in Glaucoma

Definition and measurement of I.O. Pressure, Congenital glaucoma, Chronic Simple glaucoma (Signs & treatment)

1. **Open angle glaucoma is associated with all except : AI 1993, 97**
   A. DM B. Graves disease
   C. Obesity D. Choroiditis
2. **Intra-ocular pressure is maintained by a centre in : Delhi 1993, 2000**
   A. Midbrain B. Pons
   C. Hypothalamus D. Medulla
3. **Treatment of choice for congenital glaucoma is : Delhi 1992**
   A. Drugs B. Goniotomy
   C. Trabeculotomy D. Trabeculectomy
4. **Secondary glaucoma is commonly due to : Delhi 1992**
   A. Steroids B. Ptecarpine
   C. Cataract D. Iridocyclitis
5. **100 days glaucoma is seen in : Delhi 1992**
   A. Central retinal A° occlusion
   B. Central retinal V° occlusion
   C. Neovascular glaucoma
   D. Steroid induced glaucoma
6. **The cause of glaucoma in Struge-Weber syndrome is : AIIMS 1986, 88**
   A. Occluded anterior chamber angle
   B. Swelling of the lens
   C. Angioma of the choroid
   D. Increased aqueous production
   E. Involvement of the central nervous system
7. **The volume of aqueous in the ant. chamber is : AIIMS 1988**
   A. 0.01 ml B. 0.10 ml
   C. 0.25 ml D. 0.50 ml
   E. 0.75 ml
8. **In a case of acute attack of glaucoma, Vogt's triad excludes : AIIMS 1997**
   A. Lens atrophy B. Pigment deposition
   C. Goniosynchesis D. Glaucoma fleeting
9. **The dose of Diamox (acetazolamide) in treatment of glaucoma is : AMC 1990**
   A. 100 mg every 6 hours
   B. 500 mg every 6 hours
   C. 100 mg every 24 hours
   D. 125 to 500 mg orally every 12 hours
   E. 125 to 500 mg orally every 24 hours
10. **Fincham's test is used to : AIIMS 1984, 85**
    A. Diagnose congenital glaucoma.
    B. Diagnose acute congestive glaucoma.
    C. Differential diagnose acute congestive glaucoma from cataract.
    D. Diagnose congenital cataract.
11. **Open angle glaucoma is seen in all except : AIIMS 1985**
    A. Hypertension B. Diabetes mellitus
    C. Thyrotoxicosis D. Central vein thrombosis
12. **Acute congestive glaucoma in comparison to uveitis has differences in : AIIMS 1985, 87**
    A. Size and shape of pupil
    B. Tension
    C. Type of congestion
    D. All of the above
13. **What is not the cause of glaucoma with new vascularization : AIIMS 1987, 88**
    A. Eale's disease
    B. Central retinal vein thrombosis
    C. Central retinal artery thrombosis
    D. Rubeosis Iridis

Ans. 1. D 2. C 3. C 4. A 5. B 6. C 7. C 8. A 9. D 10. C
11. A 12. D 13. C

14. Secondary glaucoma associated with angle recession is seen with : AIIMS 1994

A. Penetrating injuries B. Concussion injury
C. Radiation injury D. Chemical injury

15. Neovascular glaucoma follows : MAHE 1998

A. Thrombosis of central retinal vein
B. Acute congestive glaucoma
C. Staphylococcal infection
D. Diabetes mellitus

16. Pain in Absolute glaucoma is best relieved by : JIPMER 1992

A. Analgesics
B. Retrobullar injection of alcohol
C. Trabeculotomy
D. Miotics

17. Secondary glaucoma following perforation of cornea is caused by : JIPMER 1992

A. Angle disruption
B. Anterior synechiae formation
C. Intra ocular haemorrhage
D. Extensive peripheral synechiae

18. Which of the following is not true of Acute angle closure glaucoma : AIIMS 1992

A. Diminition of vision of rapid
B. Tension may reach upto 70 mm Hg
C. Initial instillation of Pilocarpine is useful
D. Peripheral iridectomy is contraindicated

19. The gonioscopic findings in simple glaucoma include all, except : Delhi 1984, 87

A. Changes in the trabeculae
B. Characteristic features in iris root
C. Open angle throughout the course of disease
D. Closed angle with elevated tension

20. Treatment of Open angle glaucoma is : JIPMER 1993; TN 1993

A. Iridectomy B. Atropine
C. Steroids D. Pilocarpine

21. Glaucoma capsular occurs due to : AIIMS 1986

A. Extracapsular cataract extraction
B. Intracapsular cataract extraction
C. Needling
D. Exfoliation of superficial layers of the lens capsule
E. All of the above

22. Glaucoma occurs in : Kerala 1996

A. Retinal detachment B. Vitreous degeneration
C. Myopia D. Cataract
E. Keratoconus

23. The mechanisms for causation of chronic simple glaucoma may be all except : AIIMS 1983

A. Vascular ischaemia
B. Obstruction of venous drainage.
C. Trabecular sclerosis and pigment deposit.
D. Over production of aqueous.
E. Inferrence of aqueous drainage by Schlemm's canal mechanism.

24. Early features of chronic simple glaucoma include all except : PGI 1986

A. Mild headache
B. Acute onset
C. Frequent change of presbyopic glasses
D. Blurred vision
E. Clear cornea

25. Treatment of bullous keratopathy with absolute glaucoma includes all, except : AIIMS 1984

A. Conjunctival flap
B. Corneo-scleral trephination
C. Dehydrating agents
D. Retrobulbar alcohol injection
E. Sulfonamide ointment

26. Secondary glaucoma due to angle closure is treated by all, except : BHU 1985

A. Miotics
B. Intravenous urea
C. Mydriatics
D. Carbonic anhydrase inhibitors
E. Prednisone for the control of inflammation

27. Most common associated congenital anomaly with buphthalmos is : Rajasthan 1994

A. Congenital Rubella B. Marfan's syndrome
C. Neurofibromatosis D. Lowe's syndrome

28. In a patient with intraocular lens cause of glaucoma is : CMC 1998

A. Epithelialisation of ant. chamber
B. - production of aquous
C. Secondary infection
D. Pressure of IOL

29. Secondary glaucoma in Iridocyclitis is caused by following except : Rajasthan 1995

A. Occlusio pupil B. Seclusio Pupil
C. Cyclitic membrane D. Posterior synechiae

30. Early signs of glaucoma include the following except : PGI 1997

A. Nerve fibre atrophy and haemorrhagic spots
B. Perimetric halo
C. Vertical cupping
D. None of the above

Ans.									
14. B	15. A	16. B	17. B	18. D	19. D	20. D	21. D	22. D	23. A
24. B	25. B	26. C	27. C	28. A	29. D	30. A			

31. **When there is intumescence of the lens causing glaucoma :** **TN 1987**
A. Trephining should be done
B. Paracentesis is indicated
C. Lens should be extracted
D. Glaucoma should be treated medically

32. **Malignant glaucoma may :** **AMC 1984; PGI 1999**
A. Occur in narrow angle eyes.
B. Need lens extraction.
C. Occur when surgery is performed during high tension.
D. Be prevented by pre-operative urea and mannitol.
E. All of the above

33. **Commonest presenting feature of a patient with open angle glaucoma is :** **DNB 1989**
A. Eye aches
B. Coloured haloes
C. Headaches
D. Chronic deterioration of vision noticed suddenly

34. **Intraocular pressure :** **MAHE 1996**
A. Is normally <21 mm H2O.
B. Is often raised in patients with essential systemic hypertension.
C. Is raised when the pupils are dilated in normal subjects.
D. Becomes low when the retina is detached.

35. **Increased ocular pressure in Buphthalmos causes all of the following except :** **JIPMER 1992**
A. Stretching of sclera
B. Corneal vascularization
C. Corneal curvature prominence
D. Rupture of Descemet's membrane

36. **Treatment of choice for fellow eye in angle closure glaucoma is :** **AIIMS 1993, 94; PGI 1993**
A. Timolol B. Pilocarpine
C. Yag Laser iridectomy D. Surgical iridectomy

37. **Increased intra ocular tension is seen in following except :** **Delhi 1998**
A. Epidemic dropsy B. Branch vein occlusion
C. Malignant melanoma D. Phthisis bulbi

38. **In buphthalmos following are seen except :** **PGI 1998**
A. Subluxated lens B. Large cornea
C. Small cornea D. Big eye ball

39. **Following are field lesions in open angle glaucoma except :** **PGI 1990**
A. Arcuate scotoma
B. Bjerrum scotoma
C. Enlargement of blind spot
D. Hemianopia
E. Altitudinal abnormality

40. **For tonometry used is :** **Delhi 1989**
A. 4% xylocaine B. 3% xylocaine
C. 2% xylocaine D. 1% xylocaine

41. **In chronic simple glaucoma, the most common earliest field defect is :** **Delhi 1990; PGI 2000**
A. Arcuate field defect B. Baring of blind spot
C. Bjerrum scotoma D. Siedel's sign

42. **In acute congestive glaucoma, wrong is :** **Delhi 1986, 90**
A. Relieved during sleep
B. Increased with reading in dark
C. Relieved by iridotomy
D. Field defects are prominent

43. **Intraocular pressure increases with ——— administration.** **PGI 1984, 85**
A. d-TC B. Succinylcholine
C. Gallamine D. Pancuronium

44. **Pathognomonic in open angle glaucoma is :** **Delhi 1995**
A. Siedel Sign
B. Arcuate Sign
C. Roenne's Nasal step
D. Isolated Scotomas in Bjerrum's area

45. **Hydrophthalmos is otherwise called as :** **AP 1993**
A. Secondary glaucoma B. Closed angle glaucoma
C. Open angle glaucoma D. Buphthalmos

46. **Applanation tonometer was devised by Goldman in :** **AIIMS 1986**
A. 1952 B. 1954
C. 1959 D. 1963

47. **In early glaucomatous cupping, disc is :** **Delhi 1987**
A. Round B. Oval vertically
C. Oval horizontally D. Pinpoint

48. **Following are earliest clinical signs of infantile glaucoma except :** **AIIMS 1986**
A. Epiphora
B. Blepharospasm
C. Intolerance for ligh
D. Shallow anterior chamber

49. **In a patient with acute glaucoma the prophylactic treatment for the other eye is :** **AI 1988**
A. Peripheral iridectomy B. Schele's operation
C. Anterior sclerotomy D. Iridenclesisis

50. **Most common type of glaucoma in India is :** **Delhi 1997**
A. Chronic simple glaucoma
B. Acute congesive glaucoma
C. Lens induced glaucoma
D. Steroid induced glaucoma

Ans.									
31. C	32. E	33. D	34. A	35. B	36. C	37. D	38. C	39. C	40. A
41. B	42. D	43. B	44. B	45. D	46. B	47. B	48. D	49. A	50. A

51. **In buphthalmos operation, which is a dangerous late complication : Delhi 1994**
A. Malignant glaucoma B. Endophthalmitis
C. Retinopathy D. Detachment of choroid

52. **Neovascular glaucoma is not seen in : Delhi 1994**
A. Eales disease
B. Central retinal vein occlusion
C. Branch vein occlusion
D. Diabetes mellitus

53. **Hypersecretory glaucoma is seen in : AI 1994**
A. Neuroparalytic keratitis
B. Thyrotoxic exophthalmos
C. Horner's syndrome
D. Lid retraction

54. **Unilateral glaucoma is caused by the following except : AI 1994**
A. Infantile type B. Ac. congestive
C. Corneal ulcer D. Aphakic

55. **On tightly closing the eye, the intraocular tension is : AI 1994**
A. Increased B. Decreased
C. Normal D. None of the above

56. **The following are true of normal intraocular pressure : DNB 1989**
A. Mean intraocular pressure in humans is 15-16 mmHg for sitting.
B. Distribution of intraocular pressure in the human population is skewed.
C. Mean intraocular pressure increases with age.
D. Intraocular pressure is lowest in the morning and highest at midnight.
E. There is a consistent relationship between chronic systemic hypertension and intraocular pressure.

57. **The following conditions are associated with buphthalmos : AIIMS 1989**
A. Marfan's syndrome
B. Lowe's syndrome
C. Homocystinuria
D. Von Hippel-Lindau's syndrome
E. All of the above

58. **Miotic used in glaucoma is : Rohtak 1995**
A. Atropine B. Timolol
C. Cyclopentolate D. Sympathetic stimulant

59. **In a patient with raised intraocular pressure with corneal edema, intraocular pressure is measured by : PGI 1996**
A. Schiotz tonometer B. Goldmann tonometer
C. Applanation tonometer D. Digital tonometer

60. **Drug used in glaucoma with myopic eye is : AIIMS 1986, 90, 94; Delhi 1996**
A. Pilocarpine (2%) B. Surgical treatment
C. Steroids D. Phenylephrine

61. **In acute closed glaucoma, best treatment is : AI 1996**
A. Pilocarpine B. Trabeculectomy
C. Laser iridectomy D. Physiostigmine

62. **Lady comes with H/o Halos in evening. IOT normal, dimness of vision, disease is : AIIMS 1999**
A. Prodromal AC Congestive Glaucoma
B. Incipient cong. glaucoma
C. Chronic glaucoma
D. Epidemic dropsy

63. **A 30 years old woman with sudden right-sided painful red eye associated with nausea, vomiting and headache. The diagnosis is : PGI 1999**
A. Acute congestive glaucoma
B. Endophthalmitis
C. Eale's disease
D. Trachoma

64. **Colored halo is seen in all except : PGI 1999**
A. Open angle glaucoma B. Closed angle glaucoma
C. Cataract D. None of the above

65. **Cause for coloured halos in angle closure glaucoma : TN 1999**
A. Fluid entry into cornea B. Lenticular opacities
C. Retinal detachment D. Vitreous Haemorrhage

66. **Inheritance of congenital glaucoma : MAHE 2000**
A. AD B. AR
C. XR D. None

67. **All the following anatomical changes will predispose to primary angle closure glaucoma except : AIIMS 2000**
A. Small cornea
B. Flat cornea
C. Anterior chamber shallow
D. Short axial length of eye ball

68. **In a hypertensive patient with glaucoma which of the following is not used : AIIMS 2000**
A. Dipivefrine B. Beta blockers
C. Alpha agonist D. Laser trabeculoplasty

69. **A patient complains of evening haloes and occasional headache for some months. On examination anterior chamber of both the eyes are shallow and the intraocular pressure is normal. This condition represents what state of glaucoma : AIIMS 2000**
A. Constant instability B. Prodrome
C. Absolute D. Acute

Ans.	51. A	52. C	53. D	54. A	55. A	56. B	57. E	58. B	59. C	60. A
	61. C	62. A	63. A	64. A	65. A	66. B	67. B	68. A	69. B	

70. **A 5 yrs child presents with large cornea, lacrimation and photophobia. Diagnosis is :**
PGI 1999; AI 2001; AIIMS 2001
A. Megalocornea B. Congenital glaucoma
C. Congenital cataract D. Anterior uveitis

71. **In a patient of bronchial asthma with open angle glaucoma drug of choice is : Delhi 1995, 2001**
A. Pilocarpine drops
B. Timolol drops
C. Ipratropium bromide drops
D. Betaxolol drops

72. **The following antiglaucoma drug increases uveostleral outflow : JIPMER 2002**
A. Lanatopost B. Timolol
C. Pilocarpin D. Acetazolamide

73. **In a susceptible patient, which of the following drugs precipitate glaucoma : SGPGI 2002, 2005**
A. Phenylephrine B. Phentolamine
C. Homatropine D. Epinephrine

74. **Field's chart defects are typically seen in :**
Rajasthan 2001, 2004
A. Chronic simple glaucoma
B. Closed angle glaucoma
C. Acute congestive glaucoma
D. Late stage glaucoma

75. **You have been referred a case of open angle glaucoma. Which of the following would be an important point in diagnosing the case : AI 2002**
A. Shallow anterior chamber
B. Optic disc cupping
C. Narrow angle
D. Visual acuity and refractive error

76. **Which one of the following drugs is contraindicated in the treatment of primary glaucoma : UPSC 2003**
A. Pilocarpine B. Homatropine
C. Acetazolamide D. Timolol

77. **A 60 year old female patient had normal intraocular pressure and decreased vision. The cause is : AI 2012**
A. Absolute glaucoma
B. Acute congestive glaucoma
C. Normal tension glaucoma
D. Dislocation of lesn

Ans. 70. B 71. D 72. A 73. C 74. A 75. B 76. B 77. C

EXPLANATIONS OF GLAUCOMA

1. Ans.— D. Choroiditis
2. Ans.— C. Hypothalamus
3. Ans.— C. Trabeculotomy
4. Ans.— A. Steroids
5. Ans.— B. Central retinal V° occlusion
6. Ans.— C. Angioma of the choroid
7. Ans.— C. 0.25 ml
8. Ans.— A. Lens atrophy
9. Ans.— D. 125 to 500 mg orally every 12 hours

   It is a carbonic anhydrase inhibitor used for short term basis. Methazolamide is also used.
10. Ans.— C. Differential diagnose acute congestive glaucoma from cataract.

    It is called Emsley-Fincham test. In immature cataract, there is breaking-up of halos.
11. Ans.— A. Hypertension
12. Ans.— D. All of the above
13. Ans.— C. Central retinal artery thrombosis
14. Ans.— B. Concussion injury
15. Ans.— A. Thrombosis of central retinal vein

    Neovascular glaucoma is an intractable glaucoma resulting due to formation of neovascular membrane involving the angle of anterior chamber. Neovascularization may result due to neovascularization of iris (rubeosis iridis), retinal ischaemia due to diabetic retinopathy, CRV occlusion, sickle cell retinopathy and Eale's disease. Other rare causes are chronic intraocular inflammation, intraocular tumors, longstanding retinal detachment and CRA occlusion.
16. Ans.— B. Retrobullar injection of alcohol
17. Ans.— B. Anterior synechiae formation
18. Ans.— D. Peripheral iridectomy is contraindicated
19. Ans.— D. Closed angle with elevated tension
20. Ans.— D. Pilocarpine

    In open angle glaucoma, antiglaucoma drugs i.e. topical beta blockers (Timolol maleate - 0.25 to 0.5%; betaxolol 0.25%, Levobunolol 0.25 to 0.5% and carteolol 1% to 5%; Pilocarpine (1%, 2% or 4%), Dorzolamide (2%), Latanoprost (0.0005%), adrenergic drugs (epinephrine hydrochloride (0.5, 1 or 2%) or dipiverfrine hydrochloride (0.1%), apraclonidine (0.5%), brimonidine (0.2%), oral acetazolamide or methazolamide or in combination are used.
21. Ans.— D. Exfoliation of superficial layers of the lens capsule.

    It is also called pseudoexfoliative glaucoma, which is characterized by deposition of an amorphous grey dandruff like, material on the pupillary border, anterior lens surface, posterior surface of iris, zonules and ciliary process. Secondary open angle glaucoma is seen in 50% cases.
22. Ans.— D. Cataract
23. Ans.— A. Vascular ischaemia
24. Ans.— B. Acute onset
25. Ans.— B. Corneo-scleral trephination
26. Ans.— C. Mydriatics
27. Ans.— C. Neurofibromatosis
28. Ans.— A. Epithelialisation of ant. chamber
29. Ans.— D. Posterior synechiae

    Cyclitic membrane results due to fibrosis of exudates present behind the lens. It is a late complication of acute plastic type of iridocyclitis.
30. Ans.— A. Nerve fibre atrophy and haemorrhagic spots.
31. Ans.— C. Lens should be extracted
32. Ans.— E. All of the above

33. Ans. — D. Chronic deterioration of vision noticed suddenly.

34. Ans. — A. Is normally < 21 mm H2O

35. Ans. — B. Corneal vascularization

36. Ans. — C. Yag Laser iridectomy

37. Ans. — D. Phthisis bulbi

38. Ans. — C. Small cornea

39. Ans. — C. Enlargement of blind spot

40. Ans. — A. 4% xylocaine

41. Ans. — B. Baring of blind spot

42. Ans. — D. Field defects are prominent

43. Ans. — B. Succinylcholine

44. Ans. — B. Arcuate Sign

Small-wing shaped paracentral scotoma is the earliest clinically significant field defect. It may appear either below or above the blind spot in Bjerrum's area (an arcuate area extending above and below the blind spot to between 10° to 20° of fixation point).

45. Ans. — D. Buphthalmos

46. Ans. — B. 1954

47. Ans. — B. Oval vertically

48. Ans. — D. Shallow anterior chamber

49. Ans. — A. Peripheral iridectomy

Peripheral button hole type iridectomy is done in normal eye and in diseased eye, if no ant. synechiae are present peripheral button-hole iridectomy is done and if peripheral ant. synechiae are present, iridectomy dialysis or iridencleisis is done.

50. Ans. — A. Chronic simple glaucoma

Open angle glaucoma is about 2-times more common than closed angle.

51. Ans. — A. Malignant glaucoma

52. Ans. — C. Branch vein occlusion

53. Ans. — D. Lid retraction

Sanguinarin (obtained from seeds of argenone mexicana) is the cause. Anterior chamber remains normal and field changes are similar to chronic simple glaucoma. Miotics are of no use. Withdraw contaminated mustard oil. Anterior sclerotomy is operation of choice (if required).

54. Ans. — A. Infantile type

Chronic simple glaucoma is also usually bilateral.

55. Ans. — A. Increased

Normal IOP is 16-23 mm Hg (whereas normal tissue pressure is 2-3 mm Hg and CSF pressure in recumbent position is 7 mm Hg). Deep Respiration may produce changes by 5 mm Hg whereas individual pulse beats produce pressure changes of 1-2 mmHg. In early morning it is highest. Normal physiological variation is 5 mm Hg.

56. Ans. — B. Distribution of intraocular pressure in the human population is skewed.

57. Ans. — E. All of the above

58. Ans. — B. Timolol

59. Ans. — C. Applanation tonometer

60. Ans. — A. Pilocarpine (2%)

61. Ans. — C. Laser iridectomy

Peripheral iridectomy in glaucomatous eye and prophylactic iridectomy in other eye should be done.

62. Ans. — A. Prodromal AC Congestive Glaucoma

63. Ans. — A. Acute congestive glaucoma

64. Ans. — A. Open angle glaucoma

65. Ans. — A. Fluid entry into cornea

66. Ans. — B. AR

67. Ans. — B. Flat cornea

68. Ans. — A. Dipivefrine

It is an adrenergic drug used as 0.1% solution 1-2 times/day.

69. Ans. — B. Prodrome

70. Ans. — B. Congenital glaucoma

71. Ans. — D. Betaxolol drops

72. Ans. — A. Lanatopost

73. Ans. — C. Homatropine

74. Ans. — A. Chronic simple glaucoma

75. Ans. — B. Optic disc cupping

The earliest sign is localized constriction of central field to very small test objects.

76. Ans. — B. Homatropine

Atropinic drugs are absolutely contraindicated in individuals with a narrow iridocomeal angle-may precipitate acute congestive glaucoma. However, marked rise in intraocular tension is rare in patients with chronic simple glaucoma.

77. Ans. — C. Normal tension glaucoma

Optic nerve damage and vision loss occurs inspite of normal IOP. Normal tension glaucoma affects women more often and people with average age of 60 years.

SHORT TEXTBOOK OF PSYCHIATRY

About this Book (New Edition)

- This new book is specificially written for easy grasping of Psychiatry in a clearent, pointwise, simple and easy understandable language and is exlusively based on the ***examination oriented*** pattern.
- A list of headings important for ***Undergraduate*** and ***Postgraduate examinations*** are given at the starting
- Various ***Question Papers*** of Psychiatry from previous years of many national undergraduate examinations have been added at the end of book.
- ***Multiple Choice Questions (MCQ's)***, asked on various Undergraduate and Postgraduate Examinations have been added at the end of book
- Each chapter ends with ***important points*** enlisted in abox
- A section on the general principles of Psychiatry with a special emphasis on the Historical aspects (indian/Western), ***Symptomatology*** and Psychiatric Examination has been included.
- An updated section on Psychiatric Treatments including newer advances and list of all ***Psychotropic Drugs*** in alphabetically order (according to trade names) have been added.
- Important detailed chapters on Indian Psychiatry (Contributions of Indian Psychiatrists, Epidemiology of various disorders, National Mental Health Programme of India, Forensic Psychiatry, Indian culture bound syndromes etc).
- An important list of appendices include ***Psychiatric Glossary,*** list of ***Psychological Tests, Psychiatric Side effects of Medical Drugs*** etc.
- Useful book for various Medical Competitive and Undergraduate Examination; Civil Services Examinations
- Edited by : ***Dr. M.S. Bhatia*** (M.D., Dip. W.P.A.) an experienced teacher and examiner, associated with editing of many popular books on undergraduate and Postgraduate Examinations.

CBS Publishers & Distributors Pvt. Ltd.

NEW DELHI • BANGALORE • PUNE • CHENNAI • COCHIN (INDIA)

9

IMPORTANT TEXT OF RETINA

RETINOPATHIES

Retinopathy or benign hypretension

A. In benign hypertension, if the person is young, the retinal arteries become narrow due to hypertonus of vessles. But in elderly persons, where there are already arteriosclerotic changes, the narrowing is not so marked.

B. If the hypertension is continued long, there are changes in the arterial wall, which make the vessels pale due to increased reflection of light from the wall. These changes are due to artriosclerotic changes. In more advanced stage, the arteries appear as **copper wires** and later on **silver wires,** with sheathing. The veins become compressed at the arterio-venous crossings.

But before these extreme arteriosclerotic changes occur, flame-shaped haemorrhages and hard, white and tiny exudates appear in the retina. This stage is known as the stage of arteriosclerotic retinopathy.

Retinopathy of malignant hypertension or hypertensive retinopathy

If the malignant hypertension occurs in a young adult the retinal changes are as follows :

a) Marked narrowing of the arteries
b) Flame-shaped haemorrhages
c) Wooly exudates
d) Papilloedema to some extent

The signs in the early stage

a) Micro-aneurysm formations in the retinal capillaries which appear as tiny circular red spots.
b) Yellow waxy exudate in the retina.

The signs in the later stage

a) The micro-aneurysms rupture producing circular 'dot' or 'blot' haemorrhages in the deeper layers of the retina.
b) The exudates increase but there is no oedema of the retina or of the optic disc.
c) A branch of the retinal vein may be thrombosed producing massive retinal and vitreous haemorrhage.
d) As a result of vitreous haemorrhage, retinitis proliferans may develop.

Treatment of all the retinopathies : The treatment is to treat the cause.

DIFFERENTIAL DIAGNOSIS BETWEEN PSEUDO-GLIOMA AND RETINOBLASTOMA

	Pseudo-glioma	*Retinoblastoma*
1. Nature of the disease	1. Inflammatory in origin and it is the terminal phase of endophthalmitis	1. It is a neoplasm
2. Inflammatory	2. a. Ciliary flush b. Posterior synchia c. K.P.	2. Nil
3. Tension	3. Usually low or normal	3. High
4. Progress	4. Non-progressive	4. Progressive

(Contd....)

Treatment

a) If one eye is affected, the eye must be enucleated as soon as diagnosis is made, followed by deep X-ray therapy of the orbit.
b) In bilateral cases, that eye, with a more advanced tumour, must be enucleated. Deep X-ray for the other eye may be tried.
c) When there is a fungating growth, exenteration of the orbit has to be done i.e. removal of all the contents of the orbit including the periosteum, following by deep X-ray therapy.

LESION CONFUSED WITH RETINOBLASTOMA

1. Anomalous optic disc
2. Anterior dislocated lens with secondary glaucoma
3. Coats disease (retinal telangiectasia)
4. Coloboma of choroid and optic disc
5. Congenital corneal opacity
6. Congenital rubella syndrome (Greg syndrome)
7. Cysts in a remnant of the hyaloid artery
8. Developmental retinal cyst
9. Glioma of the retina
10. Hematoma under retinal pigment epithelium
11. High myopia with advanced chorioretinal degeneration
12. Juvenile retinoschisim
13. Juvenile xanthogranuloma (nevoxanthoendothelioma)
14. Larval granulomatosis (Toxocara canis)
15. Medullation of nerve fiber layer
16. Metastatic endophthalmitis
17. Norrie disease (atrophia oculi congenita)
18. Oligodendroglioma of the retina
19. Organization of intraocular haemorrhage
20. Persistent hyperplastic primary vitreous
21. Retinal detachment due to choroidal or vitreous haemorrhage
22. Retinal dysplasia (massive retinal fibrosis)
23. Retrolental fibroplasia
24. Retrolental membrane associated with Bloch-Sulzberger syndrome (incontinentia pigementi)
25. Rhegmatogenous and falciform retinal detachment
26. Secondary glaucoma
27. Sex-linked microphthalmia
28. Tapetoretinal degeneration
29. Trisomy 13-15 (Patau syndrome)
30. Toxoplasmosis (ocular toxoplasmosis)
31. Traumatic chorioretinitis
32. Tumors other than retinoblastoma
33. Uveitis in secondary retinal detachment
34. *'White-with pressure'* sign.

MCQ's OF RETINA

What is important in Retina

Anatomy, Eale's disease, Retinopathy (esp. in diabetes and hypertension), Fundus

1. **Visible Retinal arterial pulsation is a feature of : JIPMER 1993**
   A. CRAO B. CRBO
   C. Raised IOT D. Normal eye

2. **In retinitis pigmentosa pigmentation in the retina starts at : AIIMS 1981**
   A. Posterior pole
   B. Anterior to equator region
   C. Equatorial region
   D. The disc

3. **Fibre layer of Henle is constituted by : AIIMS 1985, 87**
   A. Oblique axons of rods
   B. Oblique axons of cones in fovea centralis
   C. Both of the above
   D. Neither of the above

4. **The earliest symptom in retinoblastoma is : AP 1993**
   A. Strabismus
   B. Poor vision
   C. Proptosis
   D. Leucokoria (cat's eye reflex)

5. **Cause of retinal vein occlusion is : Delhi 1996**
   A. Neurosyphilis B. Diabetes mellitus
   C. Aplastic anaemia D. Thalassemia

6. **Retinal detachment means : WB 1996**
   A. Cleavage between layer of rods and cones from pigment epithelium
   B. Cleavage in outer portion of retina only
   C. Cleavage in inner portion of retina only
   D. All of the above

7. **In eye, - visual acquity is due to the function of : JIPMER 1996, 97**
   A. Bipolar cells B. Amacrine cells
   C. Horizontal cells D. Ganglion cells

8. **The superficial retinal haemorrhage is situated in : AIIMS 1986, 90**
   A. Nerve fibre layer B. Outer nuclear layer
   C. Inner nuclear layer D. Inner plexiform layer

9. **In K-W classification, Papilloedema is stage : AIIMS 1986, 87**
   A. I B. II
   C. III D. IV

W.10. **Salt and pepper fundus occurs in : AIIMS 1984, 90**
   A. Toxocara B. Marfan's syndrome
   C. Toxoplasma D. Rubella

11. **Earliest characteristic of diabetic retinopathy is : AI 1993; PGI 2000**
   A. A-V narrowing B. Silver wiring
   C. Microaneursyms D. Hard exudates

12. **B/L retinal detachment is seen with exudation in : JIPMER 1996**
   A. High myopia
   B. DM
   C. Optic uveitis
   D. Pregnancy induced hypertension (PIH)

13. **False about primary simple detachment of Retina is : Rajasthan 1994**
   A. Occurs at junction of retina proper & pigmentary epithelium.
   B. Due to hole in Retina.
   C. If vitreous gel is healthy such detachments rarely occur.
   D. Can be treated by Timolol drops and pad & bandage.

14. **Macula is affected in : PGI 1997**
   A. Toxoplasmosis B. CMV
   C. Malaria D. None of the above

15. **Retina is thickest at: AIIMS 1986**
   A. Disc B. Equator
   C. Ora serrata D. All have equal thickness

Ans.	1. C	2. C	3. B	4. D	5. B	6. A	7. A	8. A	9. D	10. NONE
	11. C	12. D	13. D	14. A	15. A					

16. **Retinitis pigmentosa most commonly presents as:** **AIIMS 1984, 85; UPSC 1986, 89**
A. Night blindness B. Diplobia
C. Scotoma D. Bitemporal hemianopia

17. **Blind spot in eye is:** **Delhi 1989**
A. Fovea centralis B. Macula
C. Optic disc D. None of the above

18. **Photophthalmia is caused by :** **JIPMER 1992**
A. Infrared rays B. Ultraviolet rays
C. SLE D. Trachoma

19. **All are true of Papilledema except :** **AIIMS 1992**
A. Vascular engorgement
B. Disc edema
C. Transient blurring of vision
D. Sudden painless loss of vision

20. **Bull's eye retinal lesion is seen in toxicity due to :** **AIIMS 1992**
A. Lead B. Ethambutol
C. Chloroquine D. OC Pills

21. **Which of the following is true of Diabetic retinopathy :** **AIIMS 1992; AI 1995**
A. Always associated with hypertension
B. Seen only in uncontrolled diabetes
C. Incidence increases with duration of disease
D. Determines prognosis of the disease

22. **Enlargement of blind spot is a sign of :** **JIPMER 1993**
A. Avulsion of Optic nerve
B. Papillitis
C. Papilledema
D. Retinal detachment

23. **Cattle track appearance on fundoscopy is seen in :** **Delhi 1992**
A. Central retinal-A occlusion
B. Central retinal-V occlusion
C. Syphilis
D. Diabetes mellitus

24. **All are true about retinitis circinata, except :** **AIIMS 1981**
A. It is a disease of Bruch's membrane
B. Is a cystoid degeneration of central retina
C. Shows an opaque spot in the macula
D. Shows a ring of exudate around macula
E. May show normal blood vessels

25. **Resuscitation time of the human retina following ischaemia is :** **DNB 1991**
A. 30 minutes B. 45 minutes
C. 1 to 2 hours D. 15 to 20 minutes
E. 8 minutes

26. **Findings in retinitis pigmentosa may be all of the following except :** **AIIMS 1986; PGI 2000**
A. Choroidal sclerosis and pale waxy disc
B. Night blindness
C. Increased intraocular pressure
D. Contraction of visual field and abnormal ERG
E. Retinal pigmentation resembling 'bone corpuscle'

27. **Solar retinitis is due to :** **Rohtak 1985**
A. U.V. rays B. Infrared rays
C. Retinal oedema D. Exudate in retina

28. **Retinal detachment is seen in all except :** **Kerala 1994**
A. Senile retino schisis
B. Diabetic retinopathy
C. Lattice retinal degeneration
D. Glaucoma

29. **Retina shows candle wax spots in :** **PGI 1993, 95**
A. Toxocara
B. Syphilis
C. Sarcoidosis
D. Sympathetic ophthalmitis

30. **Which of the following does not differentiate papilloedema from papillitis :** **PGI 1993, 94**
A. Disc margins are blurred
B. It is not painful
C. Vision loss is sudden
D. Vision loss is complete

31. **All of the following statements about retinitis pigmentosa are true except :** **MAHE 1996**
A. Myopia is common
B. Night blindness occurs before reading difficulties
C. Central vision is affected early
D. Cataract extraction may improve vision

32. **Which of the following is a cause of xanthopsia :** **DNB 1989**
A. Aphakia B. Cataract operation
C. Vitreous haemorrhage D. CO poisoning

33. **In chloroquine retinopathy which of the following is most useful :** **Rohtak 1987**
A. Direct ophthalmoscopy
B. Fluorescein angiography
C. Tonometry
D. ECG

34. **Separation of rods and cones due to exudative choroiditis causes :** **Rohtak 1988**
A. Photopsia B. Micropsia
C. Macropisa D. Metamorphasia

Ans.									
16. A	17. C	18. B	19. D	20. C	21. C	22. C	23. A	24. A	25. C
26. C	27. B	28. D	29. C	30. C	31. C	32. D	33. D	34. C	

35. **Microscopically the retinoblastoma : AIIMS 1986**
A. Shows calcium deposits
B. Shows cell with large hyperchromatic nuclei
C. Is composed of undifferentiated neuro-blastic cells
D. Contains numerous well-formed rosettes
E. All of the above

36. **The thickest area of the sensory retina is located in the proximity of the : AMU 1989**
A. Fovea centralis B. Optic disc
C. Equator D. Ora serrata

37. **The neuron of the second order in the retina is : Rohtak 1985**
A. Rods and cones B. Inner nuclear layer
C. Inner plexiform layer D. Outer nuclear layer
E. Ganglion cells

38. **Rhegmatogenous retinal detachment is due to : Delhi 1988**
A. Tumour B. Retinal break
C. Vitreous traction D. Proliferative retinopathy

39. **Flame shaped haemorrhages are seen in the retinopathy of : DNB 1990**
A. Diabetes B. Hypertension
C. Toxaemia D. All of the above

40. **Retinal detachment occurs in : PGI 1994**
A. Retinal vein thrombosis
B. Retinitis pigmentosa
C. Patch degeneration of retina
D. Diffuse degeneration of retina

41. **Which is a feature of exudative retinal detachment : PGI 1994**
A. Young adults B. Idiopathic
C. Sudden blindness D. All of the above

42. **One of the following is a differentiating point between retinoblastoma and pseudoglioma : AI 1995**
A. Multifocal origin
B. Calcification in retina
C. Enlargement of optic foramen
D. Low intracular pressure

43. **Retinal detachment is seen in all of the following except : AP 1994**
A. Aphakia B. Trauma
C. Uveitis D. Myopia

44. **Treatment of choice for CMV retinitis is : PGI 1994, 95**
A. Zidovidine B. Acyclovir
C. Vidarabine D. None of the above

45. **Unilateral Papilloedema with optic atrophy on the other side comprises : DNB 1990**
A. Devic's syndrome
B. Weber's syndrome
C. Foster-Kennedy syndrome
D. Laurence-Moor-Biedl syndrome

46. **In Coats' disease, the fundus findings include : AMC 1982**
A. Retinal detachment
B. Vascular dilatation
C. Anastomoses between vessels
D. Haemorrhages
E. All of the above

47. **Treatment of retinal haemangiomas may include all, except : DNB 1983**
A. Light coagulation
B. Surgical excision
C. Puncture diathermy
D. Irradiation for large diffuse lesions
E. Surface diathermy

48. **Most significant risk factor in retinal vein branch occlusion is : Delhi 1997**
A. Hypertension B. Diabetes mellitus
C. Hyperlipidemia D. Leukaemia

49. **Eale's disease is best treated with: Delhi 1990**
A. Antitubercular drugs
B. Steroids
C. Antibiotic drops
D. Antibiotics systematically

50. **Best treatment for proliferative retinopathy: Delhi 1990**
A. Argon laser
B. Krypton laser
C. Panretinal photocoagulation
D. Scleral buckling operation

51. **Commotio retinae is seen in : PGI 1984, 89**
A. Concussion injury
B. Papilloedema
C. Central vein thrombosis
D. Central artery thrombosis

52. **The following about retinoblastoma is true except : AIIMS 1984**
A. Autosomal dominant
B. Treatment is enclueation
C. Radiotherapy is also given
D. Evisceration is the treatment

53. **Retinal detachment is diagnosed by : Delhi 1985**
A. Holes B. Haemorrhage
C. Dark foreign bodies D. Headache

Ans.										
	35. E	36. B	37. E	38. C	39. B	40. B	41. D	42. D	43. C	44. A
	45. C	46. E	47. B	48. A	49. B	50. C	51. A	52. D	53. A	

54. **Simple retinal detachment is usually due to :** **AIIMS 1982, 89**
A. Tumour
B. Choroidal haemorrhage
C. Exudative retinitis
D. None of the above

55. **A type of pigmentary retinopathy may be associated with which of the following, except :** **PGI 1983**
A. Gargoylism (Hurler's syndrome)
B. Syphilis
C. Steatorrhea
D. Macroglobulinaemia
E. Rubella's syndrome

56. **Which one of the following findings is the most useful in the diagnosis of early pleurocephalic oedema (papilloedema of intracranial hypertension) :** **PGI 1984**
A. Transient amaurosis
B. Enlargement of blind spot
C. Blurred disc margins
D. Loss of venous right reflex
E. Leakage of flourescein from disc capillaries on angiography

57. **Following are indications for panretinal laser photocoagulation in diabetic retinopathy except :** **Delhi 1997**
A. Focal maculopathy
B. Preretinal haemorrhage
C. Neovascular glaucoma
D. More than 10 cotton wool spots

58. **Non-rhegmatogenous retinal detachment secondary to spontaneous uveal effusion :** **PGI 1985; Delhi 1989**
A. Is characteristically accompanied by panuveitis.
B. May be accompanied by choroidal detachment.
C. Is unilateral more often than bilateral.
D. Occurs in women more frequently than in men.
E. Characteristically extends to the ora serrata.

59. **Consider the following statements :** **UPSC 1998**
Cherry red spot of the macula is seen in
1 Tay Sach's disease
2. Sandhoff disease
3. Niemann-Pick disease
4. Generalised gangliosides.
Of these statements
A. 1 alone is correct
B. 2 and 4 are correct
C. 1, 2, 3 and 4 are correct
D. 1, 2 and 3 are correct

60. **Cherry red macula is seen in :** **Delhi 1985, 86, 87; AIIMS 1997**
A. Acute Congestive glaucoma
B. Uveitis
C. Central retinal artery occlusion
D. Central retinal vein occlusion

61. **Normal A : V ratio of fundus is :** **Delhi 1985, 87**
A. 1 : 2
B. 2 : 3
C. 3 : 2
D. 3 : 4

62. **IV layer of retina is :** **DNB 1989**
A. Layer of pigment epithelium
B. External limiting membrane
C. Outer nuclear layer
D. Outer plexiform layer

63. **The number of rods are approximately :** **AMU 1986**
A. 7 million
B. 30 million
C. 70 million
D. 120 million

64. **The aim of the treatment in retinal detachment is :** **AIIMS 1984; PGI 1986; AI 1989**
A. Drainage of subretinal fluid
B. Encirclage
C. Repair of defect
D. Stitch the retina in place

65. **Which is not found in papilloedema :** **AIIMS 1986; AI 1989**
A. Blurred vision
B. Blurred margins of disc
C. Cupping of disc
D. None

66. **Ophthalmic artery is a branch of :** **Delhi 1987**
A. Common carotid artery
B. External carotid artery
C. Internal carotid artery
D. Basilar artery

67. **Retinal change specific in proliferative diabetic retinopathy is :** **Delhi 1994**
A. Microaneurysm
B. Soft cotton wool exudate
C. A-V shunt
D. Neovascularization

68. **Treatment of retinal detachment in a patient with aphakia is :** **Delhi 1994**
A. Encircling
B. Photocoagulation
C. Buckling
D. Localized uyopexy

69. **Commonest lesion which hinders vision in diabetic retinopathy is :** **Delhi 1994**
A. Macular oedema
B. Microaneurysm
C. Retinal haemorrhage
D. Retinal detachment

70. **All of the following are seen in hypertensive retinopathy except :** **AI 1994**
A. Generalized arteriolar spasm
B. Focal arteriolar spasm
C. CSR
D. Exudates

Ans.									
54. D	55. D	56. E	57. D	58. B	59. C	60. C	61. B	62. C	63. D
64. B	65. C	66. C	67. D	68. A	69. A	70. C			

71. **The following are recognized features of retinoblastoma except : AIIMS 1984**
A. Autosomal dominant inheritance
B. Cytology characterized by mulberry collections of cells
C. Cytological staining with S100 stain
D. Homer-Wright rosettes
E. Flexner-Wintersteiner rosettes

72. **All are features of Eales disease except : AI 1994**
A. Common in young males
B. Vitreous haemorrhage
C. Optic neuritis
D. Good central vision

73. **In papilloedema correct is : AI 1994**
A. Transient loss of vision
B. Inflammatory oedema of optic disc
C. Brain tumor is commonest cause
D. Blindspot is reduced

74. **Submacular fluid can originate from all except : AI 1994**
A. The choroidal circulation
B. Incompetent retinal capillaries
C. Dysfunctioning RPE cells
D. Abnormal papillary vessels and optic nerve architecture
E. The vitreous

75. **The primary aim in retinal detachment surgery is : MP 1998**
A. Closure of the break
B. Encirclage
C. Drainage of subretinal fluid
D. Removal of vitreous

76. **Causes of cystoid macular oedema include all except : AIIMS 1982**
A. Inherited B. Adrenaline
C. Irvine-Gas syndrome D. Acetazolamide
E. Retinitis pigmentosa

77. **'Bull's eye' maculopathy is associated with all except : AIIMS 1980, 89**
A. Benign concentric annular macular dystrophy
B. Batten's ceroi-lipofuscinosis
C. Retinitis pigmentosa
D. Chloroquine
E. Cone dystrophy

78. **The following are recognized causes of cellophane maculopathy or macular pucker except : PGI 1985, 87**
A. Dysthyroid ophthalmopathy
B. Retinal detachment surgery
C. Trauma
D. CRVO
E. Extensive pan-retinal photocoagulation

79. **Causes of exudative retinal detachment include all except : DNB 1990**
A. Eclampsia B. CMV retinitis
C. Dysthyroid eye disease D. Scleritis
E. Hypoproteinemia

80. **Causes of retinal detachment in the young include all except : PGI 1986**
A. Retinoblastoma B. Eales' disease
C. Tuberous sclerose D. von-Hippel's disease
E. Coats's disease

81. **Central retinal vein occlusion is associated with the following except : DNB 1991**
A. Renal failure B. Optic nerve drusen
C. Oestrogen D. Multiple myeloma
E. Idiopathic thrombocytopenia

82. **Macular oedema is caused by following except : PGI 1998**
A. Microaneurysm B. Neovascularization
C. Capillary dilatation D. None

83. **Diabetic retinopathy is seen in : AIIMS 1998**
A. NIDDM 2 years duration
B. IDDM 2 years duration
C. Juvenile DM till puberty
D. Gestational DM

84. **Amacrine cells arise from : Kerala 1998**
A. Outer nuclear layer B. Outer plexiform layer
C. Inner plexiform layer D. Inner nuclear layer

85. **Features of papilloedema are all except : AI 1995**
A. Headache
B. Blurring of disc margin
C. Transient loss of vision
D. Sudden painfull loss of vision

86. **Black pigment along veins and waxy talling in fundoscopy suggests : AIIMS 1999**
A. Retinitis pigmentosa B. Retinal detachment
C. Diabetic retinopathy D. Retinoblastoma

87. **All of the following are true about X-ray findings in retinoblastoma except : AIIMS 1999**
A. Widening of optic canal
B. Involvement of cranial bone
C. Intraocular calcification
D. Secondaries in optic nerve

Ans. 71. C 72. C 73. C 74. C 75. B 76. D 77. C 78. A 79. C 80. C 81. E 82. B 83. C 84. D 85. D 86. A 87. B

88. A patient with systolic murmur with H/O sudden vision loss O/E anti. chamber clear, Perception of light +, cherry red spot, disease is : AIIMS 1999
A. CRAO
B. Choroiditis with SABE
C. Anterior inf. ischemic optic neuropathy
D. CRVO

89. Enlarging dot sign in fundus fluorescin scanning is seen in : PGI 1999
A. Cystoid macular edema
B. Central serous retinopathy
C. Significant macular edema
D. Coat's disease

90. Knudson's 2 step hypothesis is for : PGI 1999
A. Buphthalmos B. Glaucoma
C. Retinoblastoma D. Cataract

91. Photopsia with floaters are seen in which type of retinal detachment : AI 2000
A. Rhegmatogenous B. Traction
C. Exudative D. Ischemic

92. In which one of the following congenital infections is retinopathy a prominent feature : UPSC 2000
A. Cytomegalovirus B. Rubella
C. Syphilis D. Toxoplasmosis

93. In retinal rein thrombosis, the typical appearance of retina is: JIPMER 2000
A. Macular oedema B. Macular haemorrhage
C. Dence opacity D. Retrobulbar neuritis

94. Snow burns are due to : IAM 2000
A. UV rays B. Infrared rays
C. Snow rays D. Cosmic rays

95. In branched retinal artery occlusion, loss of vision is due to : JIPMER 2000
A. Vitreous haemorrhage B. Retinal haemorrhage
C. Papilloedema D. Scotoma

96. Fog light appearance is seen in : Delhi 2000
A. Toxocariasis B. Toxoplasms
C. Sarcoidosis D. Congenital syphilis

97. Acute retinal necrosis is seen in infection by : Delhi 2000
A. Herpes B. HIV
C. Adenovirus D. Echovirus

98. Following are true about finding on fundus oculi examination in ecclampsia except : Delhi 2000
A. Neovascularization B. Cotton wool spots
C. Retinal pigmentation D. Arterial spasms

99. Purtscher's retinopathy is seen in : Delhi 2000
A. Chest haematoma B. Ocular haematoma
C. Head injury D. Diabetes mellitus

100. Retinopathy in neonate is due to : PGI 2000
A. Prematurity < 1500 gm B. O2 toxicity
C. Trauma D. Diabetes

101. In a patient of hypertension, exudative retinopathy is aggravated by : AIIMS 2000
A. Conn's syndrome B. Renal artery stenosis
C. Coarctation of aorta D. Takayasu's arteritis

102. Which of the following statements about commotio retinae is true : Kerala 2000
A. Also known as Berlin's oedema
B. This is a common result of a blow on the eye
C. Milk white cloudiness appears at the posterior pole
D. Sometimes the cloudiness disappears after some days
E. All of the above

103. Exudative retinopathy is found in : UP 2000, 2002
A. Corrugation retina
B. Demarcation line
C. Nerve fibre layer
D. Subepithelial (pigment epithelium)

104. Which of the following not found in diabetic retinopathy on fundus examination : AI 2001, 2005
A. Microaneurysms B. Retinal haemorrhages
C. Arteriolar dilatation D. Neovascularisation

105. Which is the best investigation for retinal detachment : Kerala 2001, 2004
A. Indirect ophthalmoscopy
B. 3D lens test
C. Direct ophthalmoscopy
D. 90 D test

106. Retinal detachment occur in all except : Rohtak 2001
A. Lattice degeneration
B. Cabblestone degeneration
C. Granular tag
D. Trauma

107. Photocoagulation of retina, which quadrant is first coagulated : JIPMER 2002
A. Temporal B. Nasal
C. Superior D. Inferior

108. Laser affects which layer of the retina : BHU 2002
A. Inner nuclear layer B. Pigment layer
C. Layer of rods & cones D. Inner plexiform layer

Ans. 88. A 89. B 90. C 91. A 92. A 93. A 94. A 95. D 96. A 97. A
98. A 99. A 100. A 101. C 102. E 103. D 104. C 105. A 106. C 107. A
108. B

109. **In a patient with AIDS chorioretinitis is typically caused by : AI 2003**
A. Cytomegalovirus
B. Toxoplasma gondii
C. Cryptococcus neoformans
D. Histoplasma capsulatum

110. **Exudative retinal detachment is seen in which of the following : JIPMER 2003**
A. Penetrating injuries
B. High myopia
C. Pre-eclampsia
D. Chorioretinal degeneration

111. **Retinitis pigmentosa would affect : MAHE 2003**
A. Rods predominantly
B. Cones predominantly
C. Both equally
D. Rods only

112. **Most common second malignancy in patients with Familial Retinoblastoma is: Karnataka 2004**
A Teratoma B Medullary carcinoma
C Osteosarcoma D Malignant melanoma

113. **Retinitis pigmentosa is associated with all except : AIIMS 2008**
A. Usher syndrome
B. Kornzweig syndrome
C. Kearns-Sayre syndrome
D. Marfan syndrome

114. **Which of the following is best to differentiate CRVO from carotid artery occlusion? AI 2009**
A. Dilated retinal vein
B. Retinal artery pressure
C. Tortuous retinal vein
D. Ophthalmodynamometry

115. **In patients with systemic hypertension, the characteristic haemorrhage seen on ophthalmoscopy is : UPSC 2011**
A. Dot haemorrhage
B. Subchoroidal haemorrhage
C. Flame-shaped haemorrhage
D. Wet sponge haemorrhage

116. **Which of the following is most radio resistant structure in retina : AIIMS 2011**
A. Pigment Epithelium
B. Bipolar cell layer
C. Layers of rods and cones
D. Ganglion cell layer

117. **Untrue about retinitis pigmentosa : DNB 2011**
A. Vision is retained till late stage
B. Central vision is lost early
C. Affects rods and cones
D. Tunnel vision may be seen

118. **True about retinoblastoma : DNB 2011**
A. Present since birth
B. Seen in older children
C. Bilateral common
D. Most common sign is strabismus

119. **Metastasis of retinoblastoma is : AI 2012**
A. Haematogenous
B. Lymphatic system
C. Direct extension
D. Optic nerve invasion

Ans. 109. A 110. C 111. A 112. C 113. D 114. D 115. C 116. D 117. B 118. A 119. C

EXPLANATIONS OF RETINA

1. Ans.— C. Raised IOT

2. Ans.— C. Equatorial region

   It is a slow degenerative disease of retina in both eyes, beginning in childhood and often resulting in blindness in middle or advanced age. The degeneration affects primarily the rods and cones, particularly the former. Macula is not affected till late.

3. Ans.— B. Oblique axons of cones in fovea centralis

4. Ans.— D. Leucokoria (cat's eye reflex)

   It is commonest malignant tumor of childhood occurring 1 in 20,000 livebirths. In 25-30% there is bilateral involvement. 94% cases are sporadic and 6% familial. It arises as malignant proliferation of immature retinal neural cells called retinoblasts.

5. Ans.— B. Diabetes mellitus

6. Ans.— A. Cleavage between layer of rods and cones from pigment epithelium.

7. Ans.— A. Bipolar cells

8. Ans.— A. Nerve fibre layer

9. Ans.— D. IV

   It is Keith and Wegner (1939) classification of hypertensive retinopathy (Grade-I is mild generalized arteriolar attenuation particularly of small branches; Grade-II is marked generalized narrowing and focal attenuation of arterioles associated with deflection of veins at AV crossings (Salu's sign); Grade III is Grade II plus copper wiring of arterioles, banking of veins distal to AV crossings (Bonnet sign) and right-angle deflection of veins (Salu's sign). Flame-shaped haemorrhages, cotton-wool spots and hard exudates are also present. Grade-IV consists of Grade-III plus silver wiring of arteriles and papilloedema).

10. Ans.— NONE

    It is found in syphilis

11. Ans.— C. Microaneursyms

12. Ans.— D. Pregnancy induced hypertension (PIH)

13. Ans.— D. Can be treated by Timolol drops and pad & bandage.

14. Ans.— A. Toxoplasmosis

15. Ans.— A. Disc

16. Ans.— A. Night blindness

17. Ans.— C. Optic disc

18. Ans.— B. Ultraviolet rays

    Photo-ophthalmia refers to occurrence of multiple epithelial erosions due to the effect of ultraviolet rays especially from 311 to 290 micron. After an interval of 4-5 hours (latent period) of exposure, there occurs desquamation of corneal epithelium. There is severe burning pain, lacrimation, photophobia, blepharospasm, swelling of palpebral conjunctiva and retrotarsal folds. Crooker's glass is used to avoid exposure. Treatment is cold compresses, antibiotic ointment, oral analgesic and a tranquilizer.

19. Ans.— D. Sudden painless loss of vision

20. Ans.— C. Chloroquine

21. Ans.— C. Incidence increases with duration of disease

22. Ans.— C. Papilledema

23. Ans.— A. Central retinal-A occlusion

24. Ans.— A. It is a disease of Bruch's membrane

25. Ans.— C. 1 to 2 hours

26. Ans.— C. Increased intraocular pressure

27. Ans.— B. Infrared rays

    All visible rays and many infrared rays pass unimpeded to the retina and these are absorbed by pigmentary epithelium; the pathological changes are produced by the resultant heating effect. The lesion is infact, a burn of the retina.

28. Ans.— D. Glaucoma

29. Ans.— C. Sarcoidosis

30. Ans.— C. Vision loss is sudden

31. Ans.— C. Central vision is affected early

32. Ans.— D. CO poisoning

33. Ans.— D. ECG

34. Ans.— C. Macropisa

35. Ans.— E. All of the above

36. Ans.— B. Optic disc

37. Ans.— E. Ganglion cells

38. Ans.— C. Vitreous traction

It is primary retinal detachment seen in 40-60 years of age, males (M :F :3:2), myopia, aphakia, retinal degeneration, trauma and senile posterior vitreous detachment.

39. Ans.— B. Hypertension

40. Ans.— B. Retinitis pigmentosa

41. Ans.— D. All of the above

42. Ans.— D. Low intracular pressure

IOP is increased (There are 4 stages : quiescent, glaucomatous, extraocular extension and stage of metastasis).

43. Ans.— C. Uveitis

44. Ans.— A. Zidovidine

45. Ans.— C. Foster-Kennedy syndrome

46. Ans.— E. All of the above

47. Ans.— B. Surgical excision

48. Ans.— A. Hypertension

49. Ans.— B. Steroids

Eales disease is an idiopathic inflammation of peripheral retinal veins characterized by recurrent vitreous haemorrhage. Treatment is oral steroids (during active inflammation) laser photocoagulation (in neovascularization) or vitreoretinal surgery (in non-resolving vitreous haemorrhage and tractional retinal detachment).

50. Ans.— C. Panretinal photocoagulation

51. Ans.— A. Concussion injury

52. Ans.— D. Evisceration is the treatment

53. Ans.— A. Holes

54. Ans.— D. None of the above

Simple retinal detachment is usually idiopathic.

55. Ans.— D. Macroglobulinaemia

56. Ans.— E. Leakage of flourescein from disc capillaries on angiography

57. Ans.— D. More than 10 cotton wool spots

58. Ans.— B. May be accompanied by choroidal detachment.

59. Ans.— C. 1, 2, 3 and 4 are correct

60. Ans.— C. Central retinal artery occlusion

61. Ans.— B. 2 : 3

62. Ans.— C. Outer nuclear layer

63. Ans.— D. 120 million

64. Ans.— B. Encirclage

An alternative treatment is to induce similar sterile choroiditis in the region of retinal hole by cryosurgery.

65. Ans.— C. Cupping of disc

In papilloedema, physiological cup is usually obliterated.

66. Ans.— C. Internal carotid artery

67. Ans.— D. Neovascularization

68. Ans.— A. Encircling

69. Ans.— A. Macular oedema

70. Ans.— C. CSR

There may be copper wire or silver wire like arteries in benign hypertension whereas in malignant type, there are flame shaped haemorrhage and wooly exudates.

71. Ans.— C. Cytological staining with S100 stain

72. Ans.— C. Optic neuritis

Also called Periphelitis of retinal veins, common in young males and is unilateral. There may be retinal haemorrhages. Symptom none but sudden defective vision in vitreous haemorrhage.

73. Ans.— C. Brain tumor is commonest cause

Ocular star, blurring of disc margin and enlargement of blind spot may be seen.

74. Ans.— C. Dysfunctioning RPE cells

75. Ans.— B. Encirclage

76. Ans.— D. Acetazolamide

77. Ans.— C. Retinitis pigmentosa

78. Ans.— A. Dysthyroid ophthalmopathy

79. Ans.— C. Dysthyroid eye disease

80. Ans.— C. Tuberous sclerose

81. Ans.— E. Idiopathic thrombocytopenia

82. Ans.— B. Neovascularization

83. Ans. — C. Juvenile DM till puberty

84. Ans. — D. Inner nuclear layer

85. Ans. — D. Sudden painfull loss of vision

It is not painfull.

86. Ans. — A. Retinitis pigmentosa

87. Ans. — B. Involvement of cranial bone

88. Ans. — A. CRAO

89. Ans. — B. Central serous retinopathy

90. Ans. — C. Retinoblastoma

91. Ans. — A. Rhegmatogenous

It is a type of simple detachment.

92. Ans. — A. Cytomegalovirus

93. Ans. — A. Macular oedema

94. Ans. — A. UV rays

95. Ans. — D. Scotoma

96. Ans. — A. Toxocariasis

97. Ans. — A. Herpes

98. Ans. — A. Neovascularization

99. Ans. — A. Chest haematoma

100. Ans. — A. Prematurity < 1500 gm

101. Ans. — C. Coarctation of aorta

102. Ans. — E. All of the above

103. Ans. — D. Subepithelial (pigment epithelium)

104. Ans. — C. Arteriolar dilatation

Microaneurysms appear in retinal capillaries as tiny circular red spots.

105. Ans. — A. Indirect ophthalmoscopy

Periphery of retina is best seen with indirect ophthalmoscopy.

106. Ans. — C. Granular tag

107. Ans. — A. Temporal

108. Ans. — B. Pigment layer

109. Ans. — A. Cytomegalovirus

* One of the devastating consequence of HIV infection is CMV retinitis and the patient with high risk of CMV retinitis should undergo an ophthalmologic examination every 3-6 months.

110. Ans. — C. Pre-eclampsia

111. Ans. — A. Rods predominantly

112. Ans. — C Osteosarcoma

113. Ans. — D. Marfan syndrome

114. Ans. — D. Ophthalmodynamometry

* This investigation is said to be an important diagnostic tool in carotid artery insufficiency states.

* This technique is a safe and non-vassive method to diagnose a state of decreased ophthalmic artery pressure resulting from carotid insufficiency.

115. Ans. — C. Flame-shaped haemorrhage

116. Ans. — D. Ganglion cell layers

Radioresistant Cell of Body :

Hematological

Mature hematopoitic cell (erythrocytes, neutrophil, eosinophil, basop hil, macrophages)

Musculoskeletal

Myocyte, osteocyte, mature connective tissue, mature bone & cartilage

Brain & PNS

Ganglion cells (photoreceptors in eye) : Ganglion cells are an example of highly specialized cells that have undergone extensive maturation. Opposing, a fertilized ovum is probably the least specialized and primitive human cell.

117. Ans. — B. Central vision is lost early

There is progressive vision loss by effect on rods and cones, first experience is defective dark adaptation (night blindness), then constriction of visual field (tunnel vision) and eventially loss of central vision.

118. Ans. — A. Present since birth

Repeat Question

119. Ans. — C. Direct extension

Most common mode of spread is direct invasion of optic nerve with extension into CNS.

10

IMPORTANT TEXT OF OPTIC NERVE

LESIONS OF VISUAL PATHWAYS

1. ***Lesions of the optic nerve***
   (a) Affection of the papillomacular bundle produces central scotoma.
   (b) Affection of temporal or nasal fibres of the nerve causes corresponding field defects, e.g. temporal lesion causes defect in the nasal field and vice versa.
   (c) Total lesion of the optic nerve causes total blindness due to optic atrophy.
2. ***Lesions of the optic chiasma***
   Usual field defect is bitemporal hemianopia, i.e., loss of temporal field of vision in each eye, due to the affection of the crossed fibres from the nasal half of each retina.
   Binasal hemianopia, is extremely rare. It is produced by lesions on either side of the chiasma, so that the uncrossed fibres from the temporal half of each retina are affected. In both the conditions, there is partial optic atrophy.
3. ***Lesions of the optic tract***
   The usual field defect is homonymous hemianopia, i.e. loss of nasal field of the same side and temporal field of the opposite side. Due to proximity of the crus cerebri and oculomotor nerves to the tracts, ocular palsies and hemiplegia may by associated with tract lesions. There is also partial optic atrophy.
   Right homonymous hemianopia causes difficulty in reading.
4. ***Lesions of the lateral geniculate body***
   The field defect caused by this lesion is also homonymous hemianopia.
5. ***Lesions of optic radiations***
   Lesion across the entire radiation produces homonymous hemianopic field defect. There is no optic atrophy and pupil reactions are normal.
   A lesion in the upper or lower part of the radiation produces quadrantic hemianopia in which corresponding quadrants of each field are lost.
6. ***Lesions of the visual cortex***
   If the lesion is extensive as due to thrombosis of the calcarine artery, the field defect is homonymous hemianopia with sparing of the fixation area. But if only the areas above or below the calcarine fissure are affected, quadrantic hemianopia is produced.

PSEUDO-OPTIC NEURITIS (Lesions that Mimic Optic Neuritis)

1. Central scotomas produced by expanding lesions of anterior and middle crania fossa
   A. Craniopharyngiomas
   B. Ectopic pinealomas
   C. Hodgkin disease
   D. Lymphomas
   E. Meningiomas
   F. Metastatic carcinomas
   G. Nasopharyngeal carcinomas
   H. Plasmacytoma
   I. Pituitary adenomas

2. Blurring of the disc from drusen or papilledema
3. Ischemic optic neuropathy
4. Retinal lesions that also exhibit metamorphosia, such as severe or angiospastic retinopathy
5. Tumors of disc, such as metastatic carcinoma, gliomas, neurofibromas, hematomas, and meningiomas

PSEUDOPAPILLEDEMA (May be Mistaken for Swelling of Optic Nerve)

1. Arteriovenous aneurysms (recemose aneurysms) of the retina (Wyburn-Mason syndrome)
2. Cervico-oculoacousticus syndrome
3. Drusens of optic nerve
4. Epipapillary membrane and Bergmeister papilla
5. High hyperopia or astigmatism
6. Medullated nerve fibers (opaque nerve fibers)
7. Normal variant
8. Opacities or haziness of the media, especially nuclear sclerosis of the lens
9. Optic neuritis or papillitis
10. Tortuosity and anomalous early branching of the retinal vessels.
11. Tumors of disc, such as gliomas, meningiomas, neurinomas, neurofibromas, metastatic tumor, hematoma, and sarcoid

MCQ's OF OPTIC NERVE

What is important in Optic Nerve

Anatomy, Amblyopia, Optic atrophy, Visual pathways (especially site of lesion and defect)

1. **All are true about glioma of the optic nerve, except : AIIMS 1984**
   A. Posterior synechia
   B. Glaucoma
   C. Late retinal detachment
   D. Prolonged low-grade iridocyclitis
   E. All of the above
2. **Optic nerve thickness is ——— mm. Rohtak 1995, 98**
   A. 1.5 B. 2.0
   C. 2.5 D. 3.0
3. **Second order neurons in the optic pathways are present in : JIMPER 1993**
   A. Superior colliculus
   B. Retina
   C. Medical geniculate body
   D. Lateral geniculate body
4. **Injury to optic tract produces : Delhi 1992**
   A. Homonymous hemianopia
   B. Bitemporal hemianopia
   C. Binanal hemianopia
   D. Sparing of macular vision
5. **Central artery enters the optic nerve on its lower surface —— behind the globe. DNB 1990**
   A. 15-20 mm B. 25-30 mm
   C. 40-50 mm D. 50-60 mm
6. **Commonest nerve palsy caused by an angiomatosis of the internal carotid artery is: Delhi 1983**
   A. IVth nerve palsy B. IIIrd nerve palsy
   C. VIth nerve palsy D. None of the above
7. **The extent of field of vision is smallest for which colour: UPSC 1983**
   A. White B. Yellow
   C. Blue D. Green
8. **The optic foramen is located between: Delhi 1982**
   A. Greater and lesser wings of sphenoid
   B. Greater wing and body of sphenoid
   C. Lesser wing and body of sphenoid
   D. Lesser wing of sphenoid and ethmoid
9. **The intraorbital length of optic nerve is: Delhi 1984**
   A. 1 mm B. 4-10 mm
   C. 10 mm D. 25 mm
10. **In anterior ischamic optic neuropathy the characteristic defect is: AP 1990; MAHE 1998; Karnataka 1999**
    A. Altitudinal field defect B. Central scotoma
    C. Centrocecal scotoma D. Nasal step
11. **All of the following statements regarding the oculomotor nerve are true except : UPSC 1998**
    A. It accommodates the eye
    B. It raises the upper eyelid
    C. It innervates lateral rectus
    D. It constricts the pupil
12. **The distance of macula from optic disc is: Delhi 1985, 86**
    A. 1 disk diameter B. 2 disk diameter
    C. 3 disk diameter D. 4 disk diameter
    E. 1.5 mm
13. **Blurring of disc margin is found in: AIIMS 1984**
    A. Papillitis B. Retrobulbar neuritis
    C. Tobbacco amblyopia D. All of the above
14. **In retinoblastoma presenting features may not include: TN 1989**
    A. Anisocoria B. Watering eye
    C. Double vision D. Convergent strabismus
15. **Minimum light is maximum for stimulation of: AP 1989**
    A. Peripheral part of retina
    B. Fovea centralis
    C. Paracentral part of retina
    D. Macula lutea
    E. None of the above

Ans. 1. B 2. C 3. B 4. A 5. A 6. B 7. D 8. C 9. D 10. A
11. C 12. B 13. A 14. C 15. B

16. **Nearest relation of optic nerve is:** **AIIMS 1994**
A. Int. carotid artery
B. Pituitary stack
C. Ant. communicating artery
D. Ant. choroid artery

17. **Fundus changes in malaria may include all except:** **Rohtak 1987**
A. Optic neuritis
B. Retinal detachment
C. Retinal haemorrhages
D. Macular preretinal haemorrhage

18. **The ratio of crossed to uncrossed fibres in the optic chiasma is :** **DNB 1990**
A. 75 : 25 B. 63 : 37
C. 53 : 47 D. 50 : 50

19. **In fundus, first sign of raised intracranial pressure is:** **AIIMS 1985**
A. Filling of physiological cup
B. Blurring of nasal disk
C. Dilatation of vessels
D. None of the above

20. **All horizontal movements in the eye are affected by the lesions in the:** **AIIMS 1986**
A. Pons B. Cerebellum
C. Pretecrum D. Mid brain

21. **Homonymous upper quadrant hemianopia is seen in:** **AIIMS 1987**
A. Temporal lesions B. Parietal lobe lesions
C. Pituitary tumours D. Primary optic atrophy

22. **Near vision is not affected with:** **AIIMS 1987**
A. Atropine B. Adrenaline
C. Homatrophine D. Pilocarpine

23. **In optic neuritis the best investigation to be done include:** **PGI 1985, 86**
A. Gold perimetry
B. Keratoscopy
C. Ophthalmoscopy
D. Ophthalmodynamometry

24. **In unilateral optic nerve dysfunction, the following is seen when source of light is changed from normal eye to affected eye :** **AI 1999**
A. Both pupils dilate B. Affected pupil constrict
C. Normal pupil constrict D. Both pupils constrict

25. **Bitemporal hemianopia may be due to:** **PGI 1982, 90, 99**
A. Third ventricle tumour
B. Meningioma of sella diaphragmatics
C. Calcarine cortex infarction
D. Aneurysm of basilar artery

26. **Elevation of the disc margin is seen in:** **PGI 1984**
A. Optic atrophy B. Papillitis
C. Papilloedema D. None of the above

27. **Optic disc diameter is:** **Delhi 1985, 86**
A. 1 mm B. 1.5 mm
C. 2 mm D. 3 mm

28. **Retrobulbar neuritis is seen with:** **Delhi 1988; DNB 1990**
A. Rifampicin B. Streptomycin
C. Ethambutol D. Ethionamide

29. **The phenomenon clinically known as 'sparing of macula' may be due to collateral circulation of blood from the branches of :** **CSE 1996**
A. Anterior cerebral artery and posterior cerebral artery.
B. Posterior cerebral artery and middle cerebral artery.
C. Middle cerebral artery and anterior cerebral artery.
D. Posterior cerebral artery and superior cerebral artery.

30. **Which dimension of optic chiasma is maximum:** **AIIMS 1985**
A. Transverse
B. Sagittal
C. Dorso-ventra
D. All have equal dimensions

31. **Anterior ischaemic neuropathy is seen in the cases of :** **Karnataka 1994**
A. Chronic simple glaucoma
B. Giant cell artirtis
C. Chronic iridocyelitis
D. Sarcoidosis

32. **Hemianopia, cortical blindness, amnesia and thalamic pain are associated with the occlusion of :** **UPSC 1998**
A. Anterior cerebral artery
B. Middle cerebral artery
C. Posterior cerebral artery
D. Basilar artery

33. **Optic nerve function is best studied by :** **AI 1997**
A. Ophthalmoscope B. Retinoscope
C. Perimetry D. Goniometry

34. **In optic neuritis, following are seen except :** **AIIMS 1996**
A. Headache and vomiting
B. Pain on movement of eye
C. Sudden loss of vision
D. Afferent of pupillary reflex lost

35. **In accommodation reflex, there is :** **Delhi 1996**
A. Contraction of pupil
B. Horizontal dilatation of pupil
C. Vertical dilatation of pupil
D. Any of the above

Ans. 16. B 17. B 18. C 17. B 18. C 19. C 20. D 21. A 22. B 23. A
24. A 25. B 26. C 27. B 28. C 29. B 30. B 31. B 32. C 33. C
34. A 35. A

36. **Nutritional amblyopia is characterised by : Kerala 1996**
A. Peripheral scotoma
B. Central scotoma
C. Concentric decrease in visual field
D. Ring scotoma
E. None of the above

37. **Macular degeneration is caused by : Kerala 1996**
A. Chronic alcoholism B. Smoking
C. DM D. Eale's disease

38. **Commonest cause of papilloedema is : TN 1996**
A. Space occupying lesion
B. Panophthalmitis
C. Retrobulbar neuritis
D. Retinoblastoma

39. **Match List-I (side of lesion) with List-II (Visual field defect) and select the correct answer using the codes given below the lists : UPSC 1996**

List-I	List-II
A. Optic Nerve	1. Crossed homonymous with retained macular vision
B. Optic Chiasma	2. Crossed homonymous hemianopsia
C. Optic tract	3. Bitemporal hemianopsia
D. Visual cortex	4. Unilateral blindness

Codes :

	A	B	C	D
A.	3	4	2	1
B.	4	3	2	1
C.	3	4	1	2
D.	4	3	1	2

40. **Characteristic feature of optic neuritis is : AIIMS 1993; JIPMER 1998**
A. Afferent pupillary defect
B. Papilledema
C. Diplopia
D. Efferent pupil defect

41. **Bitemporal hamianopia seen with : AI 1993**
A. Aneurysm circule of willis
B. Temporal SOL
C. Frontal SOL
D. Retinoblastoma

42. **In eye true is : MAHE 1999**
A. CSF is present in optic disc.
B. Sup. rectus supplied by trochear nerve.
C. Edinger Westphal nucleus is present in accommodation reflex pathway.
D. IOP is 16 mmHg.

43. **A 40 yr. Old woman with bilateral disc edema & increased ICT & normal CT of head, likely diagnosis is : AI 2000**
A. Hypertensive retinopathy
B. Ischemic optic neuropathy
C. Benign intracranial hypertension
D. Papilitis

44. **"Sauce & Cottage Cheese" appearance of optic disc is seen in : AI 2000**
A. Syphilis B. CMV
C. Rubella D. Toxoplasmosis

The next two items are based on the following case history. Study the same carefully and attempt the items that follow it.

A 25 year old lady suddenly developes unilateral loss of vision decreasing from 6/6 to 4/60 with ill-sustained reaction of the pupil. She complains of slight headache and some pain in the orbit when looking upward.

45. **The most likely diagnosis is : UPSC 2000**
A. Acute frontal sinusitis B. Acute iritis
C. Brain tumour D. Retrobulbar neuritis

46. **The test that would aid most in the diagnosis is : UPSC 2000**
A. X-ray of the orbit
B. Visual field determination
C. Tonometry
D. Exophthalmometry

47. **Optic neuritis is seen in all except : PGI 2000**
A. DM B. Methanol poisoning
C. Multiple sclerosis D. SLE

48. **A five-years-old child presents with mild proptosis and loss of vision of one eye. On examination direct pupillary reflex is absent and consensual reflex is present. What is the most probable diagnosis is : AIIMS 2000**
A. Retinoblastoma
B. Optic disc angioma
C. Optic nerve glioma
D. Optic sheath meningioma

49. **A boy presents two weeks after an injury to his left eye. He complains of bilateral pain and redness and watering from right eye. What is the probable diagnosis : AIIMS 2000**
A. Endophthalmitis
B. Optic neuritis
C. Sympathetic irritation
D. Sympathetic ophthalmitis

Ans. 36. B 37. A 38. A 39. B 40. A 41. A 42. C 43. C 44. B 45. D
46. B 47. A 48. B 49. D

50. **Left sided lateral gaze is affected in leasion of : AI 2001**
A. Right frontal lobe B. Right occipital lobe
C. Left occipital lobe D. Left frontal lobe

51. **Which test is not useful in optic neuritis : AI 2001**
A. ERG
B. Evoked potential Retinogram
C. Perimetry
D. Fundoscopy

52. **Vitamin-B12 deficiency is likely to cause : AI 2001**
A. Bitemporal hemianopia
B. Binasal hemianopia
C. Heteronymous hemianopia
D. Centrocecal scotoma

53. **Pupillomotor fibres of third cranial nerve travel along with : Delhi 2001**
A. Nerve to medial rectus B. Nerve to superior rectus
C. Nerve to inferior rectus D. Nerve to inferior oblique

54. **Chalky white optic disc on fundus examination is seen in following except : AI 2001**
A. Papillitis
B. Papilloedema
C. Congenital optic atrophy
D. Demyelination

55. **The most common symptom of retrobulbar neuritis is : MAHE 2001**
A. Afferent pupillary defect
B. Loss of vision
C. Pain in eyes
D. Cotton wool spots and KP's

56. **A patient with Wernicke's disease presents with hemianopic pupillary response. The most likely site of involvement is : AI 2002**
A. Optic nerve
B. Optic tract
C. Lateral geniculate body
D. Optic radiation

57. **Hereditary retinoblastomas develop the following chromosomal deletion : AI 2003**
A. 13q14 B. 13p14
C. 14p13 D. 14q13

58. **Patient with loss of direct & consensual reflex on right side & loss of direct reflex on left side, consensual preserved on left. What is the lesion : CMC 2001**
A. Left 3rd nerve palsy with left 2nd nerve normal
B. Left 3rd nerve normal with left 2nd nerve palsy
C Left 4th nerve palsy
D. Left 3rd nerve palsy

59. **Macular sparing is seen in lesions occurring in : JIPMER 2003**
A. Optic nerve B. Optic tract
C. Occipital lobe D. Lateral geniculate body

60. **All are true about visual cycle except : AI 2009**
A. Condensation of opsin with aldehyde of retinal
B. NADP is reduced
C. NAD is reduced
D. Opsin combines with retinal to form visual purple

61. **All are seen in 3rd nerve palsy except : AIIMS 2011**
A. Ptosis
B. Diplopia
C. Miosis
D. Outwards eye deviation

62. **Homonymous hemianopia is due to lesion at : DNB 2011**
A. Optic tract B. Optic nerve
C. Optic chiasma D. Retina

Ans. 50. A 51. A 52. D 53. D 54. C 55. B 56. B 57. A 58. A 59. C 60. C 61. C 62. A

EXPLANATIONS OF OPTIC NERVE

1. Ans.— B. Glaucoma
2. Ans.— C. 2.5
3. Ans.— B. Retina
4. Ans.— A. Homonymous hemianopia

   This is characterized by incongruous homonymous hemianopia associated with contralateral hemianopic pupillary reaction (Wernicke's reaction). The lesion usually leads to partial descending optic atrophy and may be associated with contralateral-III nerve palsy and ipsilateral hemiplegia.

   The causes are TB, syphilitic meningitis, tumors of optic thalamus and aneurysms of superior cerebellar or posterior cerebral arteries.
5. Ans.— A. 15-20 mm
6. Ans.— B. IIIrd nerve palsy
7. Ans.— D. Green
8. Ans.— C. Lesser wing and body of sphenoid
9. Ans.— D. 25 mm

   Optic nerve is 47-50 mm in length. (Intaocular 1mm, intraorbital 30 mm, intracanalicular 6-9 mm and intracranial 10 mm).
10. Ans.— A. Altitudinal field defect
11. Ans.— C. It innervates lateral rectus
12. Ans.— B. 2 disk diameter

    Macula lutea or yellow spot is 1-2 mm is diameter. Optic disc diameter is 1.5 mm
13. Ans.— A. Papillitis
14. Ans.— C. Double vision
15. Ans.— B. Fovea centralis
16. Ans.— B. Pituitary stack
17. Ans.— B. Retinal detachment
18. Ans.— C. 53 : 47
19. Ans.— C. Dilatation of vessels
20. Ans.— D. Mid brain
21. Ans.— A. Temporal lesions
22. Ans.— B. Adrenaline
23. Ans.— A. Gold perimetry
24. Ans.— A. Both pupils dilate
25. Ans.— B. Meningioma of sella diaphragmatics
26. Ans.— C. Papilloedema
27. Ans.— B. 1.5 mm
28. Ans.— C. Ethambutol
29. Ans.— B. Posterior cerebral artery and middle cerebral artery.
30. Ans.— B. Sagittal
31. Ans.— B. Giant cell artritis
32. Ans.— C. Posterior cerebral artery
33. Ans.— C. Perimetry
34. Ans.— A. Headache and vomiting
35. Ans.— A. Contraction of pupil
36. Ans.— B. Central scotoma
37. Ans.— A. Chronic alcoholism
38. Ans.— A. Space occupying lesion
39. Ans.— B.

A	B	C	D
4	3	2	1
40. Ans.— A. Afferent pupillary defect
41. Ans.— A. Aneurysm circule of willis

    It is due to loss of temporal field of vision of each eye.
42. Ans.— C. Edinger Westphal nucleus is present in accommodation reflex pathway.
43. Ans.— C. Benign intracranial hypertension

    This is also called Pseudotumor cerebri. It may result due to Vitamin-A intoxication, glucocorticoids, amiodarone, oral contraceptives and tetracyclines.
44. Ans.— B. CMV

    It is most common in HIV. There are greyish patches or scattered white dots, with irregular sheathing of adjacent blood vessels and vitreous clouding.

45. Ans. — D. Retrobulbar neuritis

46. Ans. — B. Visual field determination

47. Ans. — A. DM

48. Ans. — B. Optic disc angioma

49. Ans. — D. Sympathetic ophthalmitis

50. Ans. — A. Right frontal lobe

It is due to crossing of fibres.

51. Ans. — A. ERG

ERG is best used in hereditary and constitutional disorders in retina including color blindness.

52. Ans. — D. Centrocecal scotoma

Optic neuritis mainly involve the papilla, macular bundle of nerve fibres, producing pallor of the temporal half of the optic disc.

53. Ans. — D. Nerve to inferior oblique

54. Ans. — C. Congenital optic atrophy

55. Ans. — B. Loss of vision

56. Ans. — B. Optic tract

57. Ans. — A. 13q14

"Retinoblastoma"

* "MC" pediatric intraocular malignancy.
* "Second MC primary intraocular malignancy of all age groups (first is choroidal melanoma).
* 6% familial with Autosomal dominant inheritance.
* Specific genetic locus is 13q14 (i.e. Band 14 on long arm of chromosome 13)
* MC presenting (symptom) is Leukocoria (white pupil) or Amaurotic cat's eye.
* Spontaneous regression is seen in 1% of cases especially in an eye with phithisis bulbi.
* MC cause of glaucoma in patient with retinoblastoma is neovascularisation.
* MC cause of pseudoretinoblastoma is persistent Hyperplastic primary vitreous.

58. Ans. — A. Left 3rd nerve palsy with left 2nd nerve normal

59. Ans. — C. Occipital lobe

60. Ans. — C. NAD is reduced

61. Ans. — C. Miosis

Dilation of pupil (d/t unopposed action of dilator pupillae).

62. Ans. — A. Optic tract

Repeat Question.

11

IMPORTANT TEXT OF SQUINT (Strabismus)

ANATOMY OF THE EXTRA-OCULAR MUSCLES

There are six extra-ocular muscles in each eye, of which four are rectus or straight muscles and two are oblique muscles.

The four rectus muscles originate from the common annular tendon of Zinn, situated around the optic foramen at the apex of the orbit. The muscles are inserted to the sclera by flat tendons, at various distances from limbus, as follows :

a. Superior rectus—*About 8 mm*

b. Inferior rectus—*6.5 mm*

c. Medial rectus—*5.5. mm*

d. Lateral rectus—*About 7 mm*

The lines of insertions of the superior and inferior rectus muscles are convex forward and oblique.

Origin and insertion of the oblique muscles

The superior oblique : It takes its bony origin from the upper and inner margin of the optic foramen. It inserted into the upper and outer part of the sclera behind the equator.

The inferior oblique

It originates from the floor of the orbit near end of the inferior orbital margin, and then passes outwards below the inferior rectus muscle and is inserted into the outer part of the sclera behind the equator and underneath the lateral rectus muscle.

Nerve supply of the extra-ocular muscles

a) Superior oblique—by the 4th cranial nerve

b) Lateral rectus—by the 6th cranial nerve.

c) Superior, inferior and medial rectus and the inferior oblique—by the 3rd cranial nerve.

MCQ's OF SQUINT (STRABISMUS)

What is important in Squint (Strabismus)

Ocular muscles (origin, nerve supply, action), Squint (Types, Classification, Diagnosis, Treatment)

1. **Anisophoria is the condition in which the deviation of the eyeball is : AP 1990, 96**
   A. Upwards
   B. Variable according to direction of gaze
   C. Downwards
   D. Outwards
   E. Inwards
2. **In paralytic squint, deviation of eye is : AIIMS 1980, 84, 89**
   A. Upwards
   B. Inwards
   C. Outwards
   D. In different directions of gaze
3. **Secondary deviation follows : AIIMS 1986, 87, 92**
   A. Donders law B. Listing law
   C. Herring's law D. Sherrington law
4. **Treatment for concomitant squint in a child : AIIMS 1987, 95**
   A. Require surgical repair B. Orthoptic exercises
   C. Occlusion of one eye D. Use of prisms
5. **In Foville syndrome, there is palsy of : PGI 1985**
   A. Superior rectus B. Superior oblique
   C. Inferior oblique D. Lateral rectus
6. **The yoke muscle for right superior rectus is: JIPMER 1992**
   A. Left superior oblique B. Left inferior oblique
   C. Left superior rectus D. Left inferior rectus
7. **Following are features of paralytic squint except: AIIMS 1992**
   A. Amblyopia B. Abnormal head position
   C. Unequal fixation D. Vertigo
8. **Action of right superior oblique is : DNB 1990; PGI 1993; AIIMS 1997**
   A. Laevo-depression B. Laevo-elevation
   C. Dextro-depression D. Dextro-elevation
9. **Which part of orbicularis oculi is referred to as Horner's muscle: JIPMER 1993**
   A. Temporal B. Orbital
   C. Lacrimal D. Muller's muscles
10. **Hirschberg test is used to detect : Delhi 1992**
    A. Squint B. Field defects
    C. Glaucoma D. Optic atrophy
11. **In paralytic squint : Delhi 1992; AIIMS 1994**
    A. Primary deviation > secondary deviation
    B. Primary deviation < secondary deviation
    C. Primary deviation = secondary deviation
    D. None of the above
12. **The action of the inferior oblique is : Rohtak 1986**
    A. Elevation, intorsion, abduction
    B. Elevation, intorsion, adduction
    C. Depression, intorsion, adduction
    D. Depression, extorsion, abduction
    E. Elevation, extorsion, abduction
13. **Duane's retraction syndrome may be characterised by all the following except : AIIMS 1982**
    A. Supression
    B. Limitation of abduction
    C. Upshooting or down shooting of the abducted eye
    D. Narrowing of palpebral fissure in abduction
    E. Head turn
14. **Uniocular diplopia may be seen in : AMU 1986, 90**
    A. Early cataract B. Subluxated lens
    C. Congestive glaucoma D. Alcohol poisoning
15. **Normal extent of visual field for eye is about : Rohtak 1986**
    A. Upward 60°, outward more than 90°, inwards 60° and downwards 70°.
    B. Upward 40°, outward 80°, downwards 60° and inwards 60°.
    C. Upward 80°, outward 90°, downwards 45° and inwards 50°.
    D. None of the above.

Ans.	1. B	2. D	3. C	4. B	5. D	6. B	7. A	8. A	9. D	10. A
	11. B	12. E	13. D	14. B	15. A					

16. Homonymous diplopia is due to palsy of ——— rectus. **Delhi 1992**

A. Medial B. Lateral
C. Superior D. Inferior

17. Internal ophthalmoplegia is seen in : **DNB 1990**

A. Migraine B. Infants
C. Diabetes mellitus D. Ethambutol toxicity

18. Physiologic diplopia may be produced by an object placed : **AMU 1986**

A. On the Horoptor
B. In the Panum's area
C. Within the Panum's area
D. Beyond the Panum's area
E. C+D

19. Commonest cause of diplopia is: **DNB 1990**

A. Acute congestive glaucoma
B. Head injury
C. Ocular muscle palsy
D. Diabetes mellitus

20. In a child, squint is associated with all except : **AIIMS 1996**

A. Diplopia B. Confusion
C. Stereopsia D. Vertigo

21. A 12° alternating divergent squint which becomes latent for near vision in a patient aged 30 : **Delhi 1983**

A. Is related to convergence insufficiency.
B. Should be treated with prisms.
C. Should be operated on only for cosmetic reasons.
D. Is likely to cause troublesome diplopia following surgery.
E. Should be corrected with bilateral rectus recessions.

22. Oculomotor nerve palsy features include all, except : **Rohtak 1987**

A. Facial weakness B. Divergent strabismus
C. Dilated fixed pupil D. Absent accommodation

23. The amplitude of accommodative convergence is : **AMU 1987**

A. Altered by weak cycloplegics
B. Altered by lenses & prisms
C. Decreased in older people
D. Altered by orthoptics

24. Which rectus muscle has shortest tendon : **DNB 1996**

A. Superior B. Inferior
C. Medial D. Vertigo

25. Most uncommon type of latent strabismus is : **DNB 1990**

A. Esophoria B. Exophoria
C. Hyperphoria D. Cyclophoria
E. None of the above

26. In a case of unilateral convergent squint a medial rectus recession of 5 mm will correct about : **AIIMS 1981**

A. 4° of squint B. 6° of squint
C. 8° of squint D. 12° of squint
E. 17° of squint

27. Internal ophthalmoplegia is : **Kerala 1996**

A. Paralysis of extra ocular muscles
B. Paralysis of levator palpebrae superioris
C. Paralysis of intra-ocular muscles
D. Loss of accommodation
E. None of the above

28. Under certain conditions monocular diplopia may be caused by which of the following except : **PGI 1984**

A. Peripheral iridectomy
B. Third nerve palsy
C. Retinal detachment
D. Dislocated lens
E. Treatment of eccentric fixation

29. Concommitant squint is distinguished from paralytic squint by all of the following except : **AIIMS 1987**

A. The angle of the squint is in all cardinal directions.
B. There is no limitations of ocular movement.
C. Head tilting is rare.
D. Diplopia is rare.
E. The angle of deviation depends upon which eye is fixing.

30. Bacterial toxin that may cause paralytic squint : **AIIMS 1981**

A. Staphylococcal entertroxin
B. Tetanus toxin
C. Lipopolysaccharide of Gram negative bacilli
D. Diphtheria toxin

31. Which of the following extraocular muscle has sympathetic innervation : **AP 1997**

A. Levator palpebrae Superior
B. Muller's muscle
C. Superior rectus
D. Inf. rectus

32. In right lateral rectus palsy, all of the following are seen except : **AIIMS 1997**

A. Internal squint
B. Diplopia on dextroversion
C. Microphthalmos
D. Cataract

33. Uncrossed diplopia is seen in : **AIIMS 1986**

A. Esotropia B. Exotropia
C. Exophoria D. Esophoria

Ans.									
16. B	17. C	18. E	19. C	20. C	21. E	22. A	23. A	24. C	25. D
26. D	27. C	28. B	29. E	30. D	31. B	32. D	33. A		

34. Superior rectus is supplied by : Delhi 1988, 93

A. IIIrd Nerve B. IVth Nerve
C. VIth Nerve D. VIIth Nerve

35. In Anisometropia best treatment is : AIIMS 1997, 2000

A. IOL B. Contact lens
C. Prism D. Glasses

36. Bilateral upper homonymnous quadrantanopia is due to : AI 1994

A. Parietal lobe lesion B. Temporal lobe lesion
C. Pituitary tumour D. Frontal lobe lesions

37. A patient with left eye vision+1 and right eye +5, treatment given is : AI 1994

A. Partial correction B. Over correction
C. Complete correction D. No treatment

38. Squint surgery is earliest done at : AI 1994

A. Birth B. Adulthood
C. 15 years D. 5 years

39. True statement about strabismic amblyopia is : MAHE 1998

A. Patching to be done to the eye with larger refractive error.
B. Curable if diagnosed before puberty.
C. Central vision fails to develop.
D. All children 5-7 years should be screened for its presence.

40. Which is true regarding latent squint : PGI 1994

A. Clinically called tropid
B. Detected by cover-uncover test
C. Always divergent
D. Mostly associated with decreased vision

41. Brown's syndrome is characterized by all except : PGI 1984

A. Superior oblique weakness
B. Positive forced duction test
C. Spontaneous resolution
D. Abnormal head posture
E. A palpable 'click' as the superior oblique tendon passes through the trochlea

42. Muscle in the lid attached to posterior tarsal margin is : Kerala 1994

A. Mueller's muscle B. Levator palpebrae
C. Superior oblique D. Superior rectus

43. Which muscle is Intortor of eye : AIIMS 1995

A. Medial rectus B. Superior rectus
C. Inferior rectus D. Inferior oblique

44. Which is not a feature of paralytic squint : PGI 1994, 95

A. Limited movement of eyeball
B. Diplopia
C. Change in head posture
D. Decreased visual acquity very commonly

45. Following are adductors of eye except : PGI 1996

A. Inf. oblique B. Medial rectus
C. Superior rectus D. Inferior rectus

46. VI nerve palsy is associated with : AI 1997

A. Crossed diplopia B. Uncrossed diplopia
C. Binocular D. Any of the above

47. Accomodative squint can be corrected by all except : MAHE 1999

A. Spectacles B. Contact lens
C. Exercises D. Surgery

48. A woman presenting with diplopia had her eyes displaced downward and laterally. There were restricted upward and medial movements. The nerve involved is : AIIMS 1999

A. III B. IV
C. VI D. Ophthalmic

49. Down-beat nystagmus could be due to : PGI 1999

A. Cerebellar degeneration
B. Arnold-Chiari malformation
C. Optic neuritis
D. Pontine lesion

50. Viewing a stationary object is : TN 1999

A. Convergence B. Vestibular
C. Saccadic D. Pursuit

51. Indication for mioties in squint is: JIPMER 2000

A. Accomodative squint B. Paralytic squint
C. Congenital squint D. None of the above

52. Pseudoesotropia is corrected by: Rohtak 2000

A. Orthoptic exercise B. Surgery
C. Lens D. Nothing

53. Which of the following statements is not correct about microtropia : Kerala 2000

A. It is a small esotropia
B. It is a small exotropia
C. It is less than 10 prism diopters
D. Associated with amblyopia
E. Anisometropia is a common finding

54. Basanti, a 20-years-old female presents with complaints of difficulty in reading near print. On examination there is ptosis and diplopia in looking in all directions. What is the most probable diagnosis : AIIMS 2000

A. Lateral rectus palsy B. Oculomotor palsy
C. Presbyopia D. Myasthenia gravis

Ans.										
	34. A	35. A	36. B	37. A	38. D	39. C	40. B	41. A	42. B	43. B
	44. D	45. D	46. B	47. D	48. A	49. B	50. A	51. B	52. D	53. B
	54. B									

55. **Eye deviated laterally and downwards, patient unable to look-up and medially, likely nerve involved : AI 2001**

A. Trochlear B. Trigeminal
C. Oculomotor D. Abducens

56. **In which nystagmus occurs when the patient looks straight : DNB 2001**

A. Latent B. Deviational
C. Optokinetic D. Central

57. **Paralysis of 3rd, 4th, 6th nerves with involvement of ophthalmic division of 5th nerve, localizes the lesion to : AI 2005**

A. Cavernous sinus B. Apex of orbit
C. Brainstem D. Base of skull

58. **The superior oblique muscle is supplied by : AI 2005**

A. 3rd cranial nerve B. 4th cranial nerve
C. 5th cranial nerve D. 6th cranial nerve

59. **The following are used for treatment of postoperative nausea and vomiting following squint surgery in children except : AI 2005**

A. Ketamine B. Ondansetron
C. Propofol D. Dexamethasone

60. **The reciprocal inhibition of antogonistic muscle upon lateral gaze is explained by : AIIMS 2008**

A. Sherrington law
B. Hering law
C. Laplace law
D. Hick's law

61. **Tucking of inferior lid retractors is done in : DNB 2011**

A. Senile ectropion B. Divergent squint
C. Ankyloblepharon D. Ptosis

62. **Drug used in divergent squint : DNB 2011**

A. Miotics B. Mydriatrics
C. Steroids D. Antibiotics

63. **Paralytic squint, true is : DNB 2011**

A. Diplopia
B. Tunnel vision
C. Vitreous haemorrhage
D. Floaters

Ans. 55. C 56. C 57. A 58. B 59. A 60. A 61. A 62. A 63. A

EXPLANATIONS OF SQUINT (STRABISMUS)

1. Ans.— B. Variable according to direction of gaze
2. Ans.— D. In different directions of gaze
3. Ans.— C. Herring's law
4. Ans.— B. Orthoptic exercises
5. Ans.— D. Lateral rectus
6. Ans.— B. Left inferior oblique

Movement (Yoke muscle)	*Right Eye Synergist antagonist*	*Ipsilateral (yoke muscle)*	*Left Eye Synergist (contralateral)*	*Antagonist*
Laevoversion	MR	LR	LR	MR
Dextroversion	LR	MR	MR	LR
Dextroelevation	SR	IT	IO	SO
Dextrodepression	IR	SR	SO	IO

* Laevoelevation & laevodepression are similar

7. Ans.— A. Amblyopia
8. Ans.— A. Laevo-depression
   Superior oblique is supplied by IV cranial nerve. Its main action is depression and subsidiary actions are abduction and intorsion.
9. Ans.— D. Muller's muscles
10. Ans.— A. Squint
11. Ans.— B. Primary deviation < secondary deviation
12. Ans.— E. Elevation, extorsion, abduction
13. Ans.— D. Narrowing of palpebral fissure in abduction.
14. Ans.— B. Subluxated lens
15. Ans.— A. Upward 60°, outward more than 90°, inwards 60° and downwards 70°.
16. Ans.— B. Lateral
17. Ans.— C. Diabetes mellitus
18. Ans.— E. C+D
19. Ans.— C. Ocular muscle palsy
20. Ans.— C. Stereopsia
21. Ans.— E. Should be corrected with bilateral rectus recessions.
22. Ans.— A. Facial weakness
23. Ans.— A. Altered by weak cycloplegics
24. Ans.— C. Medial
   The distance of tendons from limbus of recti are — Superior rectus (8mm), inferior rectus (6.5 mm), Medial rectus (5.5 mm), and lateral rectus (7 mm).
25. Ans.— D. Cyclophoria
26. Ans.— D. 12° of squint
27. Ans.— C. Paralysis of intra-ocular muscles
28. Ans.— B. Third nerve palsy
29. Ans.— E. The angle of deviation depends upon which eye is fixing.
30. Ans.— D. Diphtheria toxin
   In diphtheria, isolated palsies are common but ophthalmoplegia externa is rare; the pupil often escapes, the ciliary muscle never.
31. Ans.— B. Muller's muscle
32. Ans.— D. Cataract
33. Ans.— A. Esotropia
34. Ans.— A. IIIrd Nerve

35. Ans. — A. IOL

36. Ans. — B. Temporal lobe lesion

37. Ans. — A. Partial correction

38. Ans. — D. 5 years

39. Ans. — C. Central vision fails to develop

40. Ans. — B. Detected by cover-uncover test

41. Ans. — A. Superior oblique weakness

Brown's superior oblique tendon sheath syndrome is a congenital ocular motility defect due to fibrous tightening of superior oblique tendon. It is characterized by limitation of elevation of eye in adduction (normal elevation in abduction) usually straight eyes in primary position and positive forced duction test on attempts to elevate eye in adduction.

42. Ans. — B. Levator palpebrae

43. Ans. — B. Superior rectus

44. Ans. — D. Decreased visual acquity very commonly

45. Ans. — D. Inferior rectus

46. Ans. — B. Uncrossed diplopia

47. Ans. — D. Surgery

48. Ans. — A. III

Homonymous diplopia occurs on looking to the paralysed side.

49. Ans. — B. Arnold-Chiari malformation

50. Ans. — A. Convergence

51. Ans. — B. Paralytic squint

52. Ans. — D. Nothing

53. Ans. — B. It is a small exotropia

54. Ans. — B. Oculomotor palsy

55. Ans. — C. Oculomotor

Optic neuritis mainly involve the papilla, macular bundle of nerve fibres, producing pallor of the temporal half of the optic disc.

56. Ans. — C. Optokinetic

57. Ans. — A. Cavernous sinus

Lesion of cavernous sinus may affect and cause paralysis of 3rd, 4th, 6th nerves with involvement of ophthalmic division of 5th nerve, as they all constitute as structures passing through it and are likely to be affeced by disease or lesion of cavernous sinus e.g. thrombosis of the sinus, rupture or aneurysm of internal carotid artery.

Structure passing through cavernous sinus :

* Internal carotid artery with sympathetic plexus via medial wall.
* Abducens nerve is just lateral to the artery.
* Opthalmic and maxillary divisions of the trigeminal nerve, are lateral and below the artery.
* Oculomotor and trochlear nerves are on its lateral wall, on the superior aspect.

58. Ans. — B. 4th cranial nerve

* The superior oblique muscle is supplied by 4th cranial nerve i.e. Trochlear nerve.
* All the extraocular muscles are supplied by 3rd (oculomotor) cranial nerve except, lateral rectus - by 6th (abductors) nerve and superior oblique - by 4th (trochlear) nerve.

To remember : ALL3 SO4 LR6

59. Ans. — A. Ketamine

Drugs used for Post-operative nausea & vomiting following squint surgery :

1 Propofol infusion plus nitrous oxide
2. Transdermal scopolamine
3. Ondansetron and Granisetron
4. Droperidol

* *Dexamethasone* is used for the prevention of post-operative nausea-vomiting, especially chemotherapy induced nausea, vomiting. It may be useful particularly when used in combination with ondansetron.
* No role of ketamine in the prevention of post-operative nausea-vomiting (ketamine increases the intragastric pressure).

Ketamine also increases intraocular pressure.

60. Ans. — A. Sherrington law

61. Ans. — A. Senile ectropion

Weiss operation and Quickert technique are used.

62. Ans. — A. Miotics

Repeat Question. Miotics are used when there is inability to focus.

63. Ans. — A. Diplopia

Repeat Question.

SHORT TEXTBOOK OF PSYCHIATRY
(Aids to Psychiatry)

About this Book (New Edition)

- This new book is specificially written for easy grasping of Psychiatry in a clearent, pointwise, simple and easy understandable language and is exlusively based on the ***examination oriented*** pattern.
- A list of headings important for ***Undergraduate*** and ***Postgraduate examinations*** are given at the starting
- Various ***Question Papers*** of Psychiatry from previous years of many national undergraduate examinations have been added at the end of book.
- ***Multiple Choice Questions (MCQ's)***, asked on various Undergraduate and Postgraduate Examinations have been added at the end of book
- Each chapter ends with ***Important points*** enlisted in abox
- A section on the general principles of Psychiatry with a special emphasis on the Historical aspects (indian/Western), ***Symptomatology*** and Psychiatric Examination has been included.
- An updated section on Psychiatric Treatments including newer advances and list of all ***Psychotropic Drugs*** in alphabetically order (according to trade names) have been added.
- Important detailed chapters on Indian Psychiatry (Contributions of Indian Psychiatrists, Epidemiology of various disorders, National Mental Health Programme of India, Forensic Psychiatry, Indian culture bound syndromes etc).
- An important list of appendices include ***Psychiatric Glossary,*** list of ***Psychological Tests, Psychiatric Side effects of Medical Drugs*** etc.
- Useful book for various Medical Competitive and Undergraduate Examination; Civil Services Examinations
- Edited by : ***Dr. M.S. Bhatia*** (M.D., Dip. W.P.A.) an experienced teacher and examiner, associated with editing of many popular books on undergraduate and Postgraduate Examinations.

CBS Publishers & Distributors Pvt. Ltd.

NEW DELHI • BANGALORE • PUNE • CHENNAI • COCHIN (INDIA)

12

IMPORTANT TEXT OF EYELIDS & LACRIMAL SAC

LACRIMAL GLAND

Anatomy—It is a serous gland, situated at the upper and outer angle of the orbit, just within the orbital margin, in a depression of the orbital plate of the frontal bone known as the fossa for the lacrimal gland.

The ducts of the lacrimal gland which are about **12** in number, pass through the palpebral lobe of the gland and open into the conjunctival sac **4-5 mm** above the upper border of the tarsal plate of the upper lid.

Accessory lacrimal glands—These are very small glands of exactly the same structure as the lacrimal gland.

There are two types :

1. *Glands of Krause*—They number about **20** in the upper lid and **8** in the lower lid, and are deeply situated within the substantia propria of the conjunctiva, near the fornix particularly on the lateral side.
2. *Glands of Wolfring*—They are few in number situated in the conjunctiva, near the upper border of the tarsal plate.

Nerve supply of the lacrimal gland

1. *Sensory supply*—By the lacrimal branch of the ophthalmic division of the **5th** nerve.
2. *Sympathetic supply*—From the carotid plexus of cervical sympathetic.
3. *Secreto-motor fibres*—These are derived from the facial nerve.

Anatomy of the lacrimal passage

1. *Lacrimal Puncta*—These are two small openings, each of which is situated on a small elevation known as lacrimal papilla, about **6 mm** from the inner canthus on each lid margin. The puncta are visible only when the lids are slightly everted.
2. *Canaliculi*—These are two in number and they start from the puncta as narrow tubular passages to end in the lacrimal sac. Each canaliculus consists of a short vertical portion about 1 to 2 mm long and a long horizontal portion, the length of which is 6-7 mm. They are lined by stratified squamous epithelium.

   The two canaliculi may open into the lacrimal sac separately or they may join to form a common canaliculus **(sinus of Mair)** before opening into the sac.
3. *Lacrimal sac*—It is about **13 mm** long vertically and **5 to 6 mm** wide, situated in the lacrimal fossa formed by the lacrimal bone end the frontal process of the maxilla.

MCQ's OF EYELIDS & LACRIMAL SAC

What is important in Eyelids & Lacrimal Sac

Eyelids (Anatomy especially glands, nerve supply, stye, Meibomian cyst, Entropion, Ectropion, ptosis, Lagophthalmos) Lacrimal Sac (Anatomy, Dacrocystitis, DCR) Dry Eye

1. **The syndrome consisting of symmetrical enlargement of Lacrimal and Salivary gland is : AIIMS 1986, 93, 99**
   A. Sjogren's syndrome
   B. Mikulicz's syndrome
   C. Sturge-Weber syndrome
   D. Vogt-Koyanagi-Harada syndrome
2. **Lagophthalmos occurs as a result of paralysis of : Karnataka 1989**
   A. 6th cranial nerve
   B. 5th cranial nerve
   C. Levator palpebrae-superioris
   D. 7th cranial nerve
3. **Most common tumor of lid is : AIIMS 1993**
   A. Basal cell Ca
   B. Malignant melanoma
   C. Angle closure glaucoma
   D. Cataract
4. **Important causes of entropion upper lid are all except : Delhi 1994**
   A. Trachoma
   B. Chemical burns
   C. Involutional
   D. Steven Johnson's syndrome
5. **Glandular structure in the eyelid include all except : AIIMS 1982, 84**
   A. Accessory lacrimal glands of Krause.
   B. Accessory lacrimal glands of Wolfring.
   C. Tarsal glands more numerous in the lower than upper lid.
   D. Sweat glands of Moll opening directly into the hair follicles.
6. **A swelling below the inner canthus of the eye is probably due to : Bihar 1998**
   A. Chronic dacrocystitis
   B. Maxillary sinusitis
   C. Cavernous sinus thrombosis
   D. Orbital cellulitis
7. **Which is not feature of chronic staphylococcal blepharitis : PGI 1994**
   A. Marginal infiltrating of cornea
   B. Hordeolum externum
   C. Phlyctenular Keratitis
   D. Mydriasis
8. **Chronic dacryocystitis should be operated upon : Orissa 1999**
   A. As soon as possible
   B. When it is complicated with corneal ulcer
   C. When there is an acute attack
   D. Only before an intraocular operation
9. **3 months old infant with watering lacrimal sac on pressing causes regurgitation of mucopus material. What is the appropriate treatment : AIIMS 1999**
   A. Dacryo cysto rhinostomy
   B. Probing
   C. Probing with syringing
   D. Massage with antibiotics upto age of 6 months
10. **Lacrimal canaliculus is lined by ——— epithelium: Rohtak 2000**
    A. Stratified squamous
    B. Pseudostratified squamous
    C. Columnar
    D. Transitional
11. **Painless lid swelling is : Kerala 2001**
    A. H. internum B. H. externum
    C. Chalazion D. None of the above
12. **Bilateral ptosis is not seen in : AI 2001**
    A. Cogenital B. Marfan's syndrome
    C. Mysthenia gravis D. Bilateral nerve palsy

Ans. 1. B 2. D 3. A 4. D 5. C 6. A 7. C 8. A 9. D 10. A 11. B 12. B

13. Most common cause of epiphora in newborn is : Rohtak 1995, 96; DNB 2001

A. Stenosed lacrimal puntum
B. Non-canalisation of nasolacrimal duct
C. Sinusitis
D. Opthalmia neonatorum

14. Pale, waxy umbilicated nodule over the eyelid is : JIPMER 2002

A. External hordeolum
B. Internal hordeolum
C. Molluscum contagiosum
D. Chalazion

15. A 60-years old man presented with watering from his left eye since one year. Syringing revealed a patent drainage system. Rest of the ocular examination was normal. A provisional diagnosis of lacrimal pump failure was made. Confirmations of the diagnosis would be by : AIIMS 2002

A. Dacryoscintiography
B. Dacrocystography
C. Pressure syringing
D. Canaliculus irrigation test

16. Blaskowicz operation is done for : Delhi 1992

A. Proptosis B. Ptosis
C. Lagophthalmos D. Entropion

17. Wheelers operation is done in : Delhi 1992

A. Ectropion B. Entropion
C. Ptosis D. None of the above

18. Esophoria is common in : Delhi 1984

A. Myopia B. Hypermetropia
C. Presbyopia D. All of the above

19. Exophoria is common in : AIIMS 1986

A. Myopia B. Hypermetropia
C. Presbyopia D. All of the above

20. The commonest tumour of the lacrimal gland is : AIIMS 1984

A. Adenoma
B. Carcinoma
C. Granuloma
D. Benign mixed tumour
E. Pleomorphic Adenocarcinoma

21. Name the condition in which there is clear irrigation about fluorescein does not leak into the nose : AIIMS 1985

A. Normal lacrimal passage
B. Blockage of lacrimal passage
C. Upper canalicular block
D. Lower canalicular block

22. The most useful technique in assessing the function of the canaliculus is : Delhi 1984

A. Dye test B. Syringing
C. Probing D. Radioscintiliography
E. Dacryocystography

23. Epiphora in facial palsy is mostly due to : DNB 1990

A. Paralytic ectripion
B. Lagophthalmos
C. Failure of lacrimal pump activity
D. Reflex hypersecretion of tear

24. Burrow's operation is done for : PGI 1995

A. Ectropion B. Entropion
C. Lateral squint D. Glaucoma

25. Whitnall's ligament is seen in : PGI 1995

A. Mueller's musle
B. Frontal muscle
C. Levator palpebrae superiors
D. Superior oblique

26. Lacrimal gland is situated in ——— angle of orbit. Rohtak 1995

A. Upper-outer quadrant B. Upper-inner
C. Lower-inner D. Lower-outer

27. The commonest cause of entropion in children is due to : UPSC 1986

A. Congenital
B. Trauma
C. Trachoma
D. Tight bandaging as after a surgical operation

28. Chronic dacrocystitis is most often caused by : Delhi 1996

A. Str. pneumoniae
B. Corynebacterium
C. Staph. aureus
D. Klebsiela pneumoniae

29. Sling surgery should be avoided in cases of ptosis with: AIIMS 1987

A. Very poor levator action
B. Poor Bells phenomenon
C. Weak mueller's muscle
D. Multiple failed surgeries

30. Surgery of choice in the cases of where multiple ptosis operations have failed and levator action is poor in : AIIMS 1984

A. Sling surgery
B. Fasanella Servat operation.
C. Levator resection
D. Skin muscle excision

Ans. 13. B 14. C 15. A 16. B 17. B 18. B 19. A 20. E 21. C 22. D
23. C 24. B 25. A 26. A 27. A 28. A 29. B 30. A

31. **The following complication is not associated with pterygium : AMU 1986**
A. Diplopia
B. Astigmatism
C. Impaired vision
D. Squamous cell carcinoma

32. **Dysthyroid myopathy shows : AMC 1984**
A. Vertical diplopia B. Ptosis
C. Lid retraction D. Conjunctival chemosis
E. All of the above

33. **Hordeolum externum is inflammation of : Delhi 1986**
A. Zeis gland B. Tarsus
C. Meibomian gland D. Lacrimal gland

34. **In viewing the lacrimal sac with contrast media which of the following is correct : DNB 1989**
A. On frontal view the sac shadow is continuous with nasolacrimal duct.
B. Absence of dilatation in lateral aspect is pathological.
C. The normal sac is not dilated.
D. The duct terminates by opening onto the middle meatus of the nose.
E. Dilatation of the sac in frontal view is pathological.

35. **Chalazion is the infection of : UPSC 1986; AIIMS 1984**
A. Meibomian glands B. Conjunctiva
C. Cornea D. Uvea

36. **Conjunctivoplasty is indicated for : AIIMS 1986**
A. Punctum eversion B. Senile entropion
C. Senile ectropion D. Cicatrical entropion

37. **Upper lid proptosis with sclerosis of orbit. Diagnosis is : AIIMS 1987**
A. Meningioma B. Glioma
C. Neurofibroma D. None of the above

38. **Bilateral proptosis in young child is caused by following except : AIIMS 1986, 87**
A. Leukemia B. Carotid Art. aneurysm
C. Retinoblastoma D. Glioma

39. **In DCR (Dacrocystic resection) operation, the opening is made at : AIIMS 1988**
A. Middle meatus B. Inf. meatus
C. Superior meatus D. Sphenoethmoidal recess

40. **Toxin being used therapeutically for Blepharospasm, cramps, tics is : NIMHANS 1996**
A. Tetanus toxin B. Tetradoxin
C. Bungarus toxin D. Botulinum toxin

41. **The lacrimal duct opens at the : PGI 1986**
A. Superior turbinate B. Middle meatus
C. Inferior meatus D. None of the above

42. **Aniridia can be associated with : AP 1993**
A. Rhabdomyosarcoma B. Wilm's tumour
C. Retinoblastoma D. Neuroblastoma

43. **Glands of Krausse are about —— in lower lid and ——— in upper lid. AIIMS 1984**
A. 4, 12 B. 6, 16
C. 8, 20 D. 10, 30

44. **Ducts of lacrimal gland are about ——— in number. Delhi 1983**
A. 6 B. 8
C. 12 D. 16

45. **Ptosis and mydriasis are seen in : Karnataka 1987**
A. Facial palsy B. Peripheral neuritis
C. Oculomotor palsy D. Sympathetic palsy

46. **The operation of pilcation of inferior lid retractors is indicated in : AI 2003**
A. Senile ectropion B. Senile entropion
C. Cicatricial entropion D. Paralytic entropion

47. **Patient with lid lag. Diagnosis is : AI 2012**
A. Thyroid opthalmopathy
B. Multiple sclerosis
C. Oculomotor nerve palsy
D. Acute glaucoma

48. **A patient has external strabismus ptosis, uniocular diplopia. There is involvement of : AI 2012**
A. Trochlear B. Oculomotor
C. Abducens D. Facial

49.. **About chalazion, true is : AI 2012**
A. Painless condition
B. Carcinoma can arise
C. Swelling of eyelid rare
D. Anhidrosis

Ans.									
31. D	32. E	33. A	34. D	35. A	36. A	37. A	38. B	39. A	40. D
41. C	42. B	43. C	44. C	45. C	46. B	47. A	48. B	49. B	

EXPLANATIONS OF EYELIDS & LACRIMAL SAC

1. Ans.— B. Mikulicz's syndrome
2. Ans.— D. 7th cranial nerve
3. Ans.— A. Basal cell Ca

   Basal cell carcinoma is commonest (95%) usually seen in elderly people and most commonly in lower lid (50%), medial canthus (25%) upper lid (10-15%) and outer canthus (5-10%).
4. Ans.— D. Steven Johnson's syndrome
5. Ans.— C. Tarsal glands more numerous in the lower than upper lid.
6. Ans.— A. Chronic dacrocystitis
7. Ans.— C. Phlyctenular Keratitis
8. Ans.— A. As soon as possible

   DCR is the operation of choice. DCT (Dacryocystectomy) is done when DCR is contraindicated. Conjunctivo-cystorhinostomy is performed in the presence of blocked canaliculi.
9. Ans.— D. Massage with antibiotics upto age of 6 months.
10. Ans.— A. Stratified squamous
11. Ans.— B. H. externum
12. Ans.— B. Marfan's syndrome
13. Ans.— B. Non canalisation of nasolacrimal duct
14. Ans.— C. Molluscum contagiosum
15. Ans.— A. Dacryoscintiography
16. Ans.— B. Ptosis

    Ptosis is graded as mild (2 mm), moderate (3mm) and severe (4mm). In Blaskowics operation, the upper lid is doubly everted over a Desmarres lid retractor. Fasanella-Servat operation, levator resection and frontalis sling operation (brow suspension) are other operations used.
17. Ans.— B. Entropion
18. Ans.— B. Hypermetropia
19. Ans.— A. Myopia
20. Ans.— E. Pleomorphic Adenocarcinoma

    Lymphoid tumors and inflammatory pseudo-tumors constitute 50% of cases; benign epithelial tumors are 25% and malignant epithelial tumors are 25%.
21. Ans.— C. Upper canalicular block
22. Ans.— D. Radioscintiliography
23. Ans.— C. Failure of lacrimal pump activity
24. Ans.— B. Entropion

    Modified Burrow's operation is used for correcting cicatricial entropion. Jaesch-Arlt operation and modified Kelssey's operations are also used.
25. Ans.— A. Mueller's musle
26. Ans.— A. Upper-outer quadrant
27. Ans.— A. Congenital
28. Ans.— A. Str. pneumoniae

    Chronic daryocystitis is caused by staphylococci, pneumococci, streptococcus and pseudomonas and rarely TB, syphilis, leprosy and rhinosporidiosis.
29. Ans.— B. Poor Bells phenomenon
30. Ans.— A. Sling surgery
31. Ans.— D. Squamous cell carcinoma
32. Ans.— E. All of the above
33. Ans.— A. Zeis gland

    External hordeolum (stye) is characterized by acute pain and is treated with hot compresses, surgical incision, antibiotics drops, antiinflammatory drugs.
34. Ans.— D. The duct terminates by opening into the middle meatus of the nose.
35. Ans.— A. Meibomian glands
36. Ans.— A. Punctum eversion
37. Ans.— A. Meningioma
38. Ans.— B. Carotid Art. aneurysm

39. Ans. — A. Middle meatus

40. Ans. — D. Botulinum toxin

But when botulinism occurs, bilateral ophthalmoplegia interna with or without ptosis typically occurs. Total ophthalmoplegia can also occur.

41. Ans. — C. Inferior meatus

42. Ans. — B. Wilm's tumour

43. Ans. — C. 8, 20

44. Ans. — C. 12

45. Ans. — C. Oculomotor palsy

46. Ans. — B. Senile entropion

* Senile entropion - Commonly used surgical techniques are as follows :
    1. Modified wheelar's operation.
    2. Bick's procedure with Reeh's modification
    3. Tucking or plication of inferior lid retractors (Jones Reeh and wobig operation).

47. Ans. — A. Thyroid ophthalmolpathy

Lid lag is also called von Graefe sign.

48. Ans. — B. Oculomotor

These are findings in III nerve palsy.

49. Ans. — B. Carcinoma can arise

Squamous cell carcinoma or sebaceous cell carcinoma can arise. Upper eyelid is more often affected.

13

IMPORTANT MISCELLANEOUS TEXT

GRAVES' DISEASE — EXTERNAL EYE SIGNS

* Ballet's sign — Complete immobility of the globe
* Boston's sign — Jerky movement of upper lid on downward gaze.
* Dalrymple's sign — Staring appearance
* Emroth's sign — Puffy swelling of lids
* Gifford's sign — Difficulty in everting upper eyelid.
* Jellineck's sign — Increased pigmentation of lids
* Joffroy's sign — Absence of forehead wrinkling on upward gaze
* Kocher's sign — Increased lid retraction with visual fixation
* Mobius sign — Difficulty in converging
* Rosenbach's sign — Tremor of closed lids
* Sainton's sign — Delayed forehead wrinkling after upward gaze
* Stellwag's sign — Weakness of fixation on lateral gaze
* von Graefe's sign — Upper lid lag on downward gaze

EMBRYOLOGY

THE DERIVATION OF OCULAR STRUCTURES FROM EMBRYONIC TISSUES

Surface ectoderm gives rise to :

* The lens
* The epithelium of the cornea
* The epithelium of the conjunctiva and the lacrimal gland.
* The epithelium of the lids and its derivatives, the cilia, the meibomian glands, and the glands of Moll and Zeiss.
* The epithelial lining of the lacrimal passages.

Neural ectoderm gives rise to :

* The retina (with its pigment epithelium).
* The epithelium covering the ciliary processes.
* The pigment epithelium covering the posterior surface of the iris.
* The spinchter and dilator pupillar muscles.
* The optic nerve (neuroglial, nervous elements and leptomeninges).
* Part of the vitreous body.

Surface and neural ectoderm gives rise to :

* Part of the vitreous and the suspensory ligament of the lens.
* The blood vessels that persist (i.e. the choroidal, the central artery of the retina, the ciliary vessels and other vessels of the orbit) as well as the hyaloid artery, the vasa hyalodea propria, and the vessels of the vascular tunic of the lens that disappear before birth.
* The sclera

* The dural sheath of the optic nerve
* The ciliary muscle
* The substantia propria of the cornea and the endothelium of its posterior surface.
* The stroma of the iris.
* The extrinsic muscles of the eye.
* The fat, ligaments, and other connective tissue structures in the orbit.
* The upper and inner walls of the orbit.
* The connective tissue of the upper lid.

Visceral mesoderm (maxillary process) below the eye gives rise to :

* The lower and outer walls of the orbit; the structures lying behind and below the eye (i.e. the alisphenoid and malar bones, and the orbital plate of the superior maxilla).
* The connective tissue of the lower lid.

OCULAR DISEASE ASSOCIATED WITH SYSTEMIC DISEASE

Systemic Infections		
Cytomegalic inclusion disease	:	Acquired-retinitis with necrosis, haemorrhages, vascular sheathing, retinal destruction Congenital-cataract, uveitis, microphthalmos, anophthalmos, uveitis, optic nerve hypoplasia, chorioretinitis.
Measles	:	Focal macular chorioretinitis, papilloedema, optic atrophy, nystagmus, cortical blindness.
Rubella	:	Congenital syndorme-cataracts, microphthalmos, salt and pepper retinopathy around macula.
Acquired immunodeficiency syndrome	:	Retina-cotton wool spots, flame-shaped haemorrhages, vascular sheathing, Kaposi's sarcoma of lid or conjunctiva, Cytomegalovirus retinits.
Syphilis	:	Acquired-iris interstitial keratitis, salt and pepper' retinopathy, uveitis, Argyll-Robertson pupils, optic atrophy.
Histoplasmosis	:	Presumed ocular histoplasmosis syndrome-multifocal choroidal scars, peripapillary chorioretinal atrophy, haemorrhagic disciform maculopathy, linear streaks of chorioretinal atrophy Candidiasis Chorioretinitis, focal vitreous exudates.
Toxocariasis	:	Chronic, destructive endophthalmitis (children 2-9 years), localised posterior pole or peripheral granuloma.
Systemic granulomas		
Sarcoidosis	:	Acute and chronic anterior uveitis (secondary cataract, glaucoma, band keratopathy), lacrimal gland involvement, conjunctival granulomas, retinopathy (periphlebitis, neovascularisation, 'candle wax' exudates, vitreous haze, choroidal granulomas, optic neuritis).
Tuberculosis	:	Anterior uveitis, choroiditis
Connective tissue disorders		
Rheumatoid arthritis	:	Keratoconjunctivitis sicca (KCS), peripheral corneal melting syndrome, nodular, diffuse or necrotising scleritis.
Systemic lupus erythematosus	:	Skin eruption involving lids, KCS, peripheral corneal melting syndrome, necrotising scleritis, hypertensive retinopathy.
Polyarteritis nodosa	:	Necrotising sclerokeratitis, choroiditis, ischaemic optic neuropathy.
Wegener's granulomatosis	:	Nodular of diffuse scleritis, marginal corneal infiltrates, obstruction of nasolacrimal duct, uveitis, retinopathy (cotton wool spots, haemorrhages and oedema).
Seronegative arthritis		
Ankylosing spondylitis	:	Acute anterior uveitis.
Reiter's disease	:	Conjunctivitis, keratitis, acute anterior uveitis.
Psoriatic arthritis	:	Conjunctivitis, acute anterior uveitis, KCS.
Behcet's Disease	:	Anterior uveitis, conjunctivitis, retinal vasculitis, massive retinal exudation, retinal vessel vasodilation.
Juvenile chronic arthritis	:	Chronic iridocyclitis, secondary cataract, band keratopathy.

(Contd....)

OCULAR DISEASE ASSOCIATED WITH SYSTEMIC DISEASE (Contd...)

Metabolic disease

Galactosaemia	:	Infantile cataract
Fabry's disease	:	Cornea verticillata, spoke-like lens opacities.
Hypercalcaemia	:	White, subepithelial deposit of calcium as band in cornea.
Wilson's disease	:	Kayser-Fleischer ring in cornea, sunflower cataract.
Cystinosis	:	Corneal crystalline deposits.
Mucopolysaccharidoses	:	Corneal opacification, retinal pigmentary degeneration, optic atrophy

SUDDEN LOSS OF VISUAL ACUITY

1. Acute congestive glaucoma
2. Brain injury
3. Brain stem arteriovenous malformations
4. Following orbital operation
5. Fracture of the lesser wing of the sphenoid bone
6. Injury to the optic nerve
7. Meningeal carcinomatosis
8. Occlusion of central retinal artery
9. Optic neuritis, papillitis, retrobulbar neuritis
10. Quinine poisoning
11. Retinal detachment
12. Temporal arteritis
13. Vitreous or retinal haemorrhage
14. Wood alcohol poisoning (methyl)

INTRAOCULAR LENSES

IOL Materials

* **Optics :** Most are made from polymethyl methacrylate (PMMA Perspex CQ). Index of refraction of PMMA is **1.49** and specific gravity is : **1.19** Foldable optics are made from either silicone, hydrogel, or acrylic.
* *Haptics :* Most are made from PMMA, P-CQ, polypropylene, or proline.
* ***Sterilization :*** Is by ethylene oxide gas. Lenses should be rinsed before insertion to rinse off any residual chemical.

IOL Power Estimation

* Crude estimate of lens power necessary to approximate emmetropia can be made by assuming an 18D IOL will restore basic refraction to plano in an emmetropic eye. If one wishes to "emmetropize" an eye then 1.25 D should be added to 18 for each diopter of hyperopia to be corrected and 1.25 D substracted from 18 per each diopter of myopia to be corrected.
* Accurate measurement of lens power necessary for desired post-operative refraction is made by obtaining ultrasonic axial length, keratometry readings, and manufacturer's estimates of post-operative AC depth and placing these measurements in various mathematical formulas or programs.
* Formulas to calculate lens powers used most frequently include Binkhorst, Sanders-Retzlaff-Fraff, and Colenbrander-Hoffer.

Common Sources of errors

* Error in axial length measurement (0.1 mm error corresponds to error in final refraction of approximately 0.25 D).
* Error in keratometry readings (0.1 error in radius measurement corresponds to error in final refraction of approximately 0.50 D).
* Error in post-operative AC depth estimates (0.1 mm error corresponds to error in final refraction of approximately 0.05-0.25 D).

13.4 OPHTHALMOLOGY

IOL Design

* There is a plethora of IOL designs; however, they can be catagorized into posterior chamber lenses, iris supporting lenses, and anterior chamber lenses
* Trends show that J-loop and C-loop posterior chamber lenses dominate the market. The variety of anterior chamber designs has decreased.

Small incision IOL

Advantages

* Insertable through smaller incision than conventional PMMA IOLs. Therefore, reduced incidence of incision-related complications and more rapid vision recovery (decreased astigmatism).

Disadvantages

* Shorter track record of foldable lens material compared to PMMA.
* More difficult to insert than conventional PMMA IOLs.

Properties of Foldable IOLs

* Silicone (Starr, AMO)
  — Refractive index : 1.42 (Starr), 1.46 (AMO)
  — Hydrophobic, moderately fragile
  — IOL design : Multipiece or single piece biconvex optic only (limits compressibility)
  — Incision size : 4.0 mm
  — Manufacturing : East molded (does not remove monomers, impurities), produces smooth optical surface, no tumbling needed.
* *Hydrogel (Alcon)*
  — Refractive index : 1. 43
  — Hydrophilic (may reduce tissue damage), very fragile
  — IOL design : Single piece only, biconvex optic only (limits compressibility)
  — Incision size : 4.0 mm
  — Manufacturing : Lathe cut (dehydrated state), hydrated to acquire full dimension
* *Acrylic (loptex, Optical Radiation Corp)*
  — Refractive index : 1.48
  — Hydrophobic, very elastic (temperature-dependent), not fragile (resists tearing)
  — IOL designs : Multipiece or single piece, biconvex or plano convex (more compressible)
  — Incision size : 3.0 to 4.0 (Ioptex)
  — Manufacturing : Lathe cut (cryogenic), impurities removed before lathing, cyotumbling required

LASERS IN COMMON USE

Argon laser blue (488 nm, ALB) and argon laser green (514 nm, ALG)

* Most commonly used laser in ophthalmology today.
* ALB and ALG : Lasers of choice for panretinal photocoagulation, direct coagulation of retinal neovascularization, some focal retinal treatments, and all anterior segment procedures.
* ALG better suited than ALB for direct treatment of microneurysms in the macula because of ALG.

Krypton laser red (647 nm)

* Damage restricted to choroid and outer retina.
* Treatment of choice for choroidal neovascular membranes in the macula.
* No absorption by the macular luteal pigment so that 85% of krypton energy passes into the choroid.
* Little energy absorbed by hemoglobin, therefore, one can safely coagulate beneath parafoveal blood vessels.
* Intraretinal fibrosis does not occur after treatment.
* Permits treatment of choroidal neovascularization even within the foveal avascular zone.

Dye laser (577 nm to 630 nm)

* Rhodamine 6G (stimulated by high powered argon laser), which pumps dye into action.
* Can selectively target individual tissue within the eye.
* Commonly used wavelengths .
  — 577 nm; excellent for photocoagulation of blood vessels and melanin, less lens scatter than argon or krypton lasers.
  — 630 nm: primary absorption by melanin in choroid and RPE, hemoglobin minimal, excellent for panretinal photocoagulation with vitreous haemorrhage present.
* Subretinal neovascularization may be best treated by dye laser using combined wavelengths 630 nm and 577 nm.

Neodymium Yag Laser (1064 nm)

* Clinical applications
  — *Posterior capsulotomy :* Provides a non-invasive technique for cutting posterior capsule of lens after opacification develops.
  — *Iridectomy :* Does not depend on pigment, therefore excellent in blue irides.
  — *Vitreous membrane* : lysis; multiple sessions often required.
* Spot size fixed at 50 nm
* HeNe (helium neon) is coaxial aiming laser that is aligned slightly anterior to YAG beam.
* Optical breakdown: Microexplosion generated by high power density.
* Plasma is an altered state of matter wherein electrons have been dissociated from their atoms.
* Photodisruption : Laser functions by creating shock wave rather than thermal effect.
* Q-switched mode (one-billonth of a second pulse) permits shorter burst (one trillonth of a sec.)

MCQ's OF MISCELLANEOUS

What is important in Miscellaneous

Nystagmus, Proptosis, Vitamin-A deficiency, Injuries, (Symp. ophthalmia), Operations, Manifestations of important Systemic Diseases, All named signs, tests and factual data etc.

1. **YAG laser is used in the treatment of: AIIMS 1992**
   A. Diabetic retinopathy B. Open angle glaucoma
   C. After cataract D. Retinal detachment
2. **Frequent change of presbyopic glasses is an early symptom of: AIIMS 1992**
   A. Closed angle glaucoma B. Open angle glaucoma
   C. Senile cataract D. After cataract
3. **Painful eye movement is a feature of : PGI 1993**
   A. Iridocyclitis B. Papilloedema
   C. Corneal ulcer D. Vernal catarrh
4. **Following peripheral iridectomy, the changes occur include except: PGI 1993**
   A. Shallow anterior chamber
   B. Choroidal degeneration
   C. Malignant glaucoma
   D. Haemorrhage
5. **Pilocarpine is not used in young adults as it causes: PGI 1993**
   A. Myopia
   B. Allergy with circumcorneal congestion
   C. Cystic blebs of iris
   D. Fatigue reaction
6. **Sudden increase in blood sugar in a diabetic causes: JIPMER 1993**
   A. Myopia B. Hypermetropia
   C. Presbyopia D. Aniosmetropia
7. **All of the following are seen in albinism except : JIPMER 1993**
   A. Glaucoma B. Refractive error
   C. Nystagmus D. Photophobia
8. **Rupture of Descemet's membrane is seen in: TN 1993**
   A. Keratoconus B. Rubella
   C. Glaucoma D. Retinoblastoma
9. **Chronic use of steroids may lead to : Delhi 1992**
   A. Iris atrophy B. Glaucoma
   C. Corneal opacity D. Retinopathy
10. **Hutchinson's rule applies to : Delhi 1992**
    A. Interstitial keratitis B. Ptosis
    C. Squint D. Herpes zoster
11. **Salmon patch appearance is seen in : Delhi 1992**
    A. Interstitial keratitis B. Injuries
    C. Wilson's disease D. Tuberous sclerosis
12. **Polychromatic luster is seen in : Delhi 1992; AIIMS 1993, 95, 96**
    A. Complicated cataract B. Diabetes mellitus
    C. Post. irridiation cataract D. Congenital cataract
13. **Munson's sign is seen in : Delhi 1992**
    A. Keratoconus B. Keratoglobus
    C. Keratomalacia D. All of the above
14. **Commonest cause of blindness in India is : Delhi 1992**
    A. Cataract B. Glaucoma
    C. Trachoma D. Vit-A deficiency
15. **Myasthenia gravis can be diagnosed using : AIIMS 1984**
    A. Prostigmine B. Atropine
    C. Glucose D. Calcium
16. **Unilateral blindness with contralateral hemiplegia is due to : PGI 1986**
    A. Frontal lobe tumor
    B. Carotid artery aneurysm
    C. Carotid artery occlusion
    D. Head injury
17. **Congenital moles are commonest : AIIMS 1985**
    A. Near limbus
    B. At outer canthus
    C. At 5 cms away from limbus
    D. On palpebral conjuctiva
    E. On fornix

Ans. 1. C 2. B 3. A 4. C 5. C 6. A 7. A 8. A 9. B 10. D
11. A 12. A 13. A 14. A 15. A 16. C 17. A

18. Earliest ocular manifestation of Vit.-A deficiency is : **AMU 1987**

A. Bitot's spot B. Keratomalacia
C. Night blindness D. Xerosis

19. Reese-Ellswort classification is used for : **AMU 1988**

A. Trachoma B. Sympathetic ophthalmia
C. Diabetic retinopathy D. Retinoblastoma

20. Contact lens of soft type has following complications except : **Delhi 1996**

A. Acanthioemeba infection
B. Folliculosis
C. Neovascularization of cornea
D. Giant cell papillary conjunctivitis

21. Nyctalopia is seen in the following except : **Delhi 1996**

A. Oguchi disease
B. Extensive chorioretinitis
C. Retinsive pigmentosa
D. Toxocariasis

22. Endothelial melanosis is seen in all of the following except : **AMU 1986**

A. Uveitis
B. Hepatolenticular degeneration
C. Turk's line
D. Krukenberg's spindle

23. Joffroy's sign is found in cases of : **AIIMS 1985**

A. Diabetes mellitus B. Marfan syndrome
C. Thyrotoxicosis D. Tay Sach's disease
E. Hypothyroidism

24. Frontal lobe lesions may cause all of the following except : **AMU 1984**

A. Exophthalmos
B. Unilateral lowering of visual acuity
C. Superior quadrantic field defect
D. Changes in corneal reflex
E. Gaze-paretic nystagmus to opposite site

25. The surgical protection of the globe in exophthalmos may be all, except : **AMU 1986**

A. Cervical sympathectomy
B. Decompression of the orbit
C. Tarsorrhaphy
D. Resection of the levator

26. Angioid streaks : **AIIMS 1986**

A. Reveals tears in Bruch's membrane
B. Are associated with macular degeneration
C. Are seen in Paget's disease
D. Are seen in Gronblad-Strandberg syndrome
E. All of the above

27. Ocular lesions in toxocara infestation may be : **AMU 1985**

A. Retinal detachment B. Secondary glaucoma
C. A cyclitic membrane D. Low grade iridocyclitis
E. All of the above

28. Leber's congenital amourosis is characterized by: **AMU 1985**

A. Zonular or complete cataract
B. Pigmentary clumping in retina
C. Reduced visual acuity
D. Normal appearing retina
E. All of the above

29. The canal of Schlemm possesses the following anatomic characteristics : **AMU 1987**

A. Contains red cells
B. Contains aqueous
C. Lined by endothelium
D. Contains partitions resembling the dural venous trabeculae
E. All of the above

30. Vortex vein drains: **JIPMER 1992**

A. Iris and ciliary body B. Sclera
C. Uveal tract D. Retina

31. The average volume of the orbit is : **AIIMS 1983**

A. 6 cc B. 12 cc
C. 18 cc D. 24 cc
E. 30 cc

32. All the following structures are located in the lateral wall of the cavernous sinus except : **AIIMS 1983**

A. Oculomotor nerve B. Trochlear nerve
C. Ophthalmic nerve D. Maxillary nerve
E. Abducens nerve

33. Distance of limbus from ora serrata in emmetropic eye is —— mm. **Rohtak 1995, 96**

A. 6 B. 8
C. 10 D. 12

34. Structures involved in the control of saccadic eye movements include all except : **AMU 1987**

A. Cerebellum B. Superior colliculus
C. Temporal cortex D. Posterior commissure
E. Medial longitudinal bundle

35. Complication of extracapsular extraction of cataract is : **Delhi 1996; AIIMS 1995**

A. Post. opacities B. Retrobulbar neuritis
C. Eale's disease D. Night blindness

36. Schwalbe's ring corresponds to : **BHU 1986**

A. Corneal endothelium B. Descemet's membrane
C. Schlemm's canal D. Ciliary body

Ans.									
18. C	19. D	20. B	21. D	22. B	23. C	24. C	25. D	26. E	27. E
28. E	29. E	30. C	31. E	32. E	33. B	34. C	35. A	36. B	

37. Pseudo-Graefe phenomenon may be found following recovery from paralysis of the : **DNB 1991**

A. Fourth cranial cerve B. Seventh cranial nerve
C. Third cranial nerve D. Sixth cranial nerve

38. All of the following are features of Ehlers Danlos syndrome, except : **AIIMS 1983**

A. Blue sclera B. Long suture
C. Subluxation of lens D. Epicanthal folds
E. Keratoconus

39. Moderate loss of vision in diabetes mellitus is due to : **Delhi 1996**

A. Vitreous haemorrhage B. Cataract
C. Exudative retinopathy D. Glaucoma

40. All the following can be seen in Axenfeld's anomaly except : **Rohtak 1985**

A. Posterior embryotoxon
B. Iris synechiae to Schwalbe line
C. Ectopic of the pupil
D. Glaucoma

41. All the following are true concerning Rieger's anomaly except : **PGI 1984**

A. Autosomal recessive inheritance.
B. Glaucoma
C. The possible presence of facial dental and osseous.
D. The spectrum of Axenfeld's anomaly and marked annulus development of the iris mesoderm.

42. Goldenhar's syndrome is associated with what prominant ocular manifestation : **AIIMS 1986**

A. Micro cornea B. Sclero cornea
C. Megalo cornea D. Epibulbar dermoids
E. Nystagmus

43. All the following are true regarding leutic interstitial keratitis except : **AIIMS 1981**

A. It generally is a bilateral diseases in the congenital form.
B. The congenital form usually present at the age 5 of or under.
C. It is associated with deafness and Hutchinson's teeth (Hutchinson's triad).
D. It is associated with anterior uveitis.

44. The most common parasitic infestation found in the orbit among following is : **Delhi 1984; PGI 1996**

A. Echinococcus granulosus
B. Cysticercus cellulosae
C. Entamoeba histolytica
D. Schistosoma hematobium

45. Photophthalmia is treated by : **Delhi 1996**

A. Corticosteroid B. Irrigation with saline
C. Beta blockers D. Surgery

46. Superior orbital fissure syndromes are frequently caused by : **AMC 1987**

A. Carotid aneurysms B. Arachnoditis
C. Meningioma D. All of the above

47. Kayser Fleisher ring is found in which layer of cornea: **PGI 1988**

A. Bowman's membrane B. Substantia propria
C. Descemet's membrane D. Endothelium

48. Following are inert foreign bodies in eye except : **DNB 1990; AI 2000; MAHE 2001**

A. Gold B. Silver
C. Copper D. Platinum

49. The following statements about persistent hyperplastic primary vitreous (PHPV) are correct except : **DNB 1990**

A. Posterior PHPV is the most common type.
B. PHPV typically occurs in an otherwise normal eye.
C. PHPV is usually bilateral.
D. Ciliary processes are abnormal.
E. Prognosis for vision is good in anterior PHPV.

50. Following are mucin-deficiency diseases except : **AIIMS 1982**

A. Vitamin-A deficiency
B. Stevens-Johnson's syndorme
C. Trachoma
D. Exposure keratopathy
E. Essential shrinkage of the conjunctiva

51. X-ray following injection of a contrast medium into the lacrimal passage shows the following except : **AIIMS 1984**

A. The naso-lacrimal duct terminates into the middle meatus.
B. The normal sac appears dilated in the PA view.
C. The PA view shows the sac to be continuous with the nasolacrimal duct.
D. The lateral view of the sac showing absence of dilatation of the sac is pathological.

52. The normal pH of tear is : **DNB 1991**

A. 5.7 B. 6.7
C. 7.5 D. 7.9
E. 8.4

53. The cause of bloody tears include following except : **DNB 1989**

A. Severe conjunctivitis B. Haemophilia
C. Jaundice D. Conjunctival granuloma
E. None of the above

Ans.									
37. C	38. B	39. A	40. C	41. A	42. D	43. B	44. A	45. B	46. D
47. C	48. C	49. D	50. D	51. C	52. C	53. E			

54. **Most common cause of ocular prolapse in children is : Delhi 2000**
A. Cavernous sinus thrombosis
B. Congenital defect
C. Retinoblastoma
D. Grave's disease

55. **The septum orbitale is pierced by all of the following except : BHU 1985**
A. The supratrochlear nerve
B. Muller's muscle
C. Supraorbital vessels and nerves
D. Lacrimal vessels and nerves
E. The levator muscle in the uppler lid

56. **Systemic diseases associated with band keratopathy include : AIIMS 1986**
A. Paget's disease B. Still's disease
C. Boeck's sarcoid D. Myotonica dystrophy
E. All of the above

57. **Which of the following is the most common ocular complication with renal transplantation : DNB 1991**
A. Cataract
B. Glaucoma
C. Cytomegalic inclusion virus retinitis
D. Candida kerato mycosis
E. Candida endophthalmitis

58. **Mydriatic with rapid cycloplegia is caused by : AI 1997**
A. Phenylephrine B. Atropine
C. Cyclopentolate D. Tropicamide

59. **Anticholinergic that is not a mydriatic is : AI 1997**
A. Cycrimine B. Pirenzepine
C. Isopropamide D. Ipratropium

60. **Artery supply of visual cortex is by —— branches of arteries. Delhi 1996**
A. Posteromedial, Post. cerebral
B. Posterolateral, Post-cerebral
C. Post. inf. cerebral
D. Anteromedial middle cerebral

61. **Which of the following is false : Delhi 1982**
A. Optokinetic nystagmus may be obtained during the first month of life.
B. Acuity of 6/9 is usual by 4 years of age.
C. Accommodation does not commence before 2 months.
D. Convergence does not commence before 2 months.
E. At 6 months the orbital axes are directed towards the nasal septum.

62. **Vossious ring is seen in : AI 1996**
A. Cornea B. Ant. Capsule of lens
C. Post. capsule of lens D. Retina

63. **Sudden loss of unilateral vision and pain on movement is seen in : AI 1996**
A. Diabetes mellitus B. Retrobulbar neuritis
C. Hypertension D. IIIrd nerve palsy

Match each glaucoma operation with one of the condition (Ques. 64 to 68) : AI 1996

64.	**Malignant glaucoma**	A.	**Cyclodialysis**
65.	**Post-operative iritis**	B.	**Trephine**
66.	**Distorted pupil**	C.	**Iridencleisis**
67.	**Late endophthalmitis**	D.	**Scheie's operation**
68.	**Hyphaema**	E.	**Preoperative narrow angle**

69. **A man of 40 presents with unilateral VI, VII, VIII and XII nerves palsies : Which one of the following is the most likely diagnosis : DNB 1991**
A. Syringobulbia
B. Thrombosis of posterior-inferior cerebellar artery
C. Disseminated sclerosis
D. Sarcoidosis
E. Nasopharyngeal carcinoma

70. **Which of the following is most likely to be the cause of a painful third nerve palsy of sudden onset in a man of 40 : AIIMS 1986**
A. Rupture of an infraclinoid aneurysm
B. Sphenoidal ridge meningioma
C. Diabetes mellitus neuropathy
D. Haemorrhage into a pituitary tumour
E. Rupture of a supraclinoid aneurysm

71. **What is chalcosis : PGI 1984**
A. Reaction due to copper of foreign body in the cornea
B. Reaction due to lime
C. Type of cataract
D. Blood staining

72. **The commonest intra-ocular tumour in children is : AMU 1986**
A. Malignant melanoma
B. Retinoblastoma
C. Teratoid medulloepithelioma
D. Diktyoma

73. **A semilunar fold of skin, situated above and sometimes covering the inner canthus is known as : Rohtak 1987**
A. Coloboma of lid B. Epicanthus
C. Cryptophthalmos D. Microblepharon

Ans.										
	54. C	55. B	56. E	57. A	58. D	59. A	60. B	61. D	62. B	63. B
	64. E	65. D	66. C	67. B	68. A	69. E	70. E	71. A	72. B	73. B

74. Fit each of the conditions (A) to (E) with one of the appearances (i) to (v) seen on plain radiography of the skull : **AIIMS 1983**

I. Chronically raised intracranial pressure	(1) Calcified foci (brain stones) scattered over the cerebral cortex
II. A tumour of the cerebral hemisphere	(2) Flecks of calcium in the subcortex and basal ganglia of the brain
III. Toxoplasmosis	(3) Erosion of the posterior clinoid processes
IV. Sturge Weber syndrome	(4) Displacement of the calcified pineal to one side
V. Tuberous sclerosis	(5) Parieto-occipital tram line calcification

A.	I (i)	II (ii)	III (iii)	IV (iv)	V (v)
B.	I (ii)	II (iii)	III (iv)	IV (v)	V (i)
C.	I (iii)	II (iv)	III (ii)	IV (v)	V (i)
D.	I (iv)	II (iii)	III (ii)	IV (i)	V (v)

75. Hyphemia is blood in the : **BHU 1996**
A. Ant. chamber B. Post. chamber
C. Cornea D. Conjunctiva

76. Sudden loss of vision in a quiet eye with a normal media and fundus may be due to : **UPSC 1996**
A. Vitreous haemorrhage
B. Iridocyclitis
C. Keratitis
D. Acute retrobulbar neuritis

77. The pathology of snow blindness involves the : **DNB 1991**
A. Cornea B. Iris
C. Retina D. All of the above

78. Herberts pits are seen on the : **AIIMS 1987**
A. Lid margin B. Palpebral conjunctiva
C. Arlt's line D. Limbus

79. Complete paralysis of extraocular muscles occur in : **AMC 1985**
A. Orbital cellulitis
B. Panophthalmitis
C. Cavernous sinus thrombosis
D. All of the above

80. Blind spot of Mariotte is : **AP 1986**
A. Fovea centralis B. Macula lutea
C. Optic Disc D. None of the above

81. Oro-oculo-genital syndrome occurs due to : **UPSC 1996**
A. Vit.-A deficiency
B. Vit.-B1 deficiency
C. Vit-B2 deficiency
D. Nicotinic acid deficiency

82. Which of the following statements are correct : **AP 1987**
A. Reverse cutting needles are not suitable for corneal suturing.
B. In keratomileusis removal of convex lens from the corneal disc will make the eye more hypermetropic.
C. Elastic fibres are absent in extraocular muscle.
D. Approximately 60 muscle fibres are supplied by each motor neurone in extraocular muscular.
E. All of the above.

83. The deposits seen in arcus senilis are : **Delhi 1983**
A. Lipid material B. Calcium salt
C. Hyaline material D. None of the above

84. Toxoplasmosis usually affects : **AIIMS 1985**
A. Iris B. Ciliary body
C. Macula D. Ora serrata

85. Expulsive haemorrhage may occur in following : **AIIMS 1985**
A. Blunt injury with hyphema
B. Perforating injury
C. Lens extraction
D. Panophthalmitis

86. The pigment deposited is Kayser-Fleischer ring is : **Delhi 1934**
A. Melanin B. Haemosiderin
C. Copper compound D. None of the above

87. Features of toxoplasmosis in children include : **Delhi 1982**
A. Presence of choroiditis since birth.
B. The earliest ocular sign is localized retinal oedema.
C. The macular lesions show iritense pigmentation.
D. The exudates cause vitreous haze.
E. All of the above.

88. In the Laurence-Moon-Biedle syndrome all of the following may be found, except : **PGI 1986**
A. Retinal detachment B. Mental retardation
C. Hypogenitalism D. Retinitis pigmentosa
E. Obesity

89. Adrenal corticosteroid therapy is contraindicated in all, except : **AIIMS 1984**
A. Small pox B. Chickenpox
C. Fungus infection D. Herpes zoster
E. Keratitis

Ans.										
	74. C	75. A	76. A	77. A	78. D	79. C	80. C	81. D	82. B	83. A
	84. C	85. C	86. C	87. E	88. A	89. D				

90. Contraindications to the use of corneal contact lenses include all of the following except : AIIMS 1983
A. Inadequate motivation
B. Esotropia
C. Inflammatory or degenerative conditions of anterior segment
D. Dusty environment condition
E. Spectacle corrections requiring prisms

91. Bowen's disease is characterized by all, except : PGI 1987
A. Predilection for the limbus
B. Poikilocarynosis
C. Presence of "monster cells"
D. Being incapable of metastasizing
E. Epithelial hyperplasia

92. Which of the following does not develop from surface ectoderm : DNB 1989
A. Corneal epithelium
B. Conjunctival epithelium
C. Ciliary epithelium
D. Lacrimal gland epithelium
E. Lens

93. Primary endothelial dystrophy of the senile type may reveal all of the following, except : AIIMS 1983
A. Diffuse stromal haze
B. Endothelial changes most marked in periphery
C. Corneal guttata
D. Endothelial changes most marked in the centre
E. Heavy diffuse endothelial pigmentation

94. Indications of enucleation include all of the following except : AIIMS 1983
A. Phthisis bulbi
B. Panophthalmitis
C. Absolute glaucoma
D. Total anterior staphyloma
E. Painful blind eye

95. Subepithelial lesions may be found in all of the following except : DNB 1989
A. Herpes zoster
B. Nummular Keratitis
C. Measles
D. Epidemic keratoconjunctivitis

96. For Rubeosis iridis, most common cause is : JIPMER 1997
A. Diabetes mellitus
B. CRAO
C. CRVO non-proliferative
D. CRVO proliferative

97. Malignant melanoma of eye commonly affects the : TN 1996
A. Sclera B. Choroid
C. Retina D. Iris

98. Sclerosis of the bony orbit is seen with : Delhi 1983
A. Neurofibroma B. Meningioma
C. Retinoblastoma D. Glioma

99. Vossious ring is : AMU 1985
A. A type of traumatic cataract
B. Ring of brown granules of pigment on anterior capsule
C. Located behind pupillary margin
D. All of the above
E. None of the above

100. Ipsilateral-III cranial nerve involvement with contralateral hemiplegia is seen in : TN 1996
A. Weber's syndrome
B. Foville's syndrome
C. Millard-Gubler syndrome
D. Benedict's syndrome

101. Synchisis scintillans is due to ——. TN 1996
A. Gold particles B. Calcium salts
C. Cholesterol crystals D. Haematin crystals

102. Appearance of eye ball is pinkish red in : AIIMS 1983
A. Episcleritis B. Phlyctena
C. Inflammed pinguecula D. All of the above
E. None of the above

103. Photophthalmia is caused by : Delhi 1987
A. β-rays B. infra red rays
C. Ultra-violet rays D. X-rays
E. None of the above

104. 'Safe zone' of the eye ball is : DNB 1990
A. At the limbus
B. 3-4 mm behind the limbus
C. 8-9 mm behind the limbus
D. 12 mm behind the limbus
E. 1 mm behind the limbus

105. Night blindness may be caused by : AIIMS 1984
A. Vit.-A deficiency B. Retinitis pigmentosa
C. Choriodermia D. Syphilis
E. All of the above

106. All are true about angioid streaks, except : AIIMS 1982; Delhi 1999
A. They are mistaken for blood vessels.
B. They are situated at a superficial level than the retinal vessels.
C. They result due to defects in Bruch's membrane.
D. They may be associated with pseudoxanthoma elasticum.

Ans.									
90. B	91. D	92. C	93. B	94. B	95. C	96. A	97. B	98. B	99. D
100. A	101. C	102. A	103. C	104. C	105. E	106. B			

107. Peripheral anterior synechia after an acute congestive attack occurs earliest in the : **AIIMS 1982**

A. Lower part B. Upper part
C. Lower and inner part D. Lower and outer part
E. Medial part

108. Hippus is seen in : **DNB 1991**

A. Optic neuritis B. Optic atrophy
C. Papilloedema D. All of the above
E. None of the above

109. All are true about uraemic amaurosis, except : **DNB 1991**

A. It is bilateral
B. Fundi show not react to light
C. Pupil does not react to light
D. The onset of blindness is sudden
E. Vision usually improves in 10-18 hours

110. Fit in each of the conditions (I) to (V) with one of the signs (i) to (v) : **AIIMS 1985**

I Basilar artery disease	(i) Intermittent twitching of one eyelid for a few hours
II Phenytoin	(ii) Oculogyric crisis intoxication
III Myokymia	(iii) Chronic intermittent twitching of one eyelid with facial weakness
IV Clonic facial spasm	(iv) Cerebellar ataxia and nystagmus
V Postencephalitic Parkinsonism	(v) Altitudinal herniaopia

A. I (i) II (ii) III (iii) IV (iv) V (v)
B. I (ii) II (i) III (iii) IV (iv) V (v)
C. I (v) II (iv) III (i) IV (iii) V (ii)
D. I (v) II (i) III (ii) IV (iii) V (iv)

111. Which of the following is not seen in Down's syndrome : **Rajasthan 1994**

A. Oblique palpebral fissures
B. Cataract
C. Epicanthic folds
D. Ectropion

112. Solar burns in eyes most commonly occurs at : **Rajasthan 1994**

A. Macula B. Cornea
C. Optic disc D. Lens

113. Ciliary ganglion injury is characterized by : **AMC 1985**

A. Mydriasis
B. Myotonic pupil
C. Unilaterality
D. Associated Adie's syndrome
E. All of the above

114. The commonest cause of the Foster-Kennedy syndrome is : **AIIMS 1984**

A. Occipital tumour
B. Frontal lobe tumour
C. Chiasmal tumour
D. Sphenoid wing meningioma
E. Meningitis

115. Ocular signs of syringomyelia include : **PGI 1983**

A. Choked disc B. Rotatory nystagmus
C. Horner's syndrome D. Primary optic atrophy
E. All of the above

116. Ring scotoma may occur in all except : **AIIMS 1986**

A. Glaucoma B. Retinitis pigmentosa
C. Optic nerve lesions D. None of the above

117. Biconvex lens is used in all, except : **AIIMS 1987**

A. Aphakia B. Presbyopia
C. Astigmatism D. Hypermetropia

118. Complete loss of vision is seen at the onset of : **AIIMS 1930**

A. Panophthalmitis
B. Orbital cellulitis
C. Cavernous sinus thrombosis
D. All of the above

119. Stony hard eye is seen in : **Kerala 1990**

A. Infantile glaucoma
B. Acute congestive glaucoma
C. Chronic simple glaucoma
D. Absolute glaucoma
E. None of the above

120. Which of the following may be the cause of leucocoria in a child under the age of 4 except : **AMU 1985**

A. Coats disease
B. Persistent primary hyperplastic vitreous
C. Juvenile xanthogranuloma
D. Norrie's disease
E. Metastatic endophthalmitis

121. Light coagulation may be used in all except : **Delhi 1989**

A. In the treatment of retinoblastoma, seeds 6 mm diameter.
B. In the treatment of angiomatosis retinae.
C. In the treatment of central serous retinopathy.
D. In the treatment of malignant melanoma of choroid.
E. In the treatment of updrawn pupil.

Ans.									
107. B	108. E	109. C	110. C	111. D	112. A	113. E	114. D	115. E	116. D
117. C	118. A	119. D	120. C	121. A					

122. Most important complication of traumatic hyphema is: **CMC 1990**

A. Iridocyclitis
B. Iridodialysis
C. Blood staining of cornea
D. Siderosis bulbi

123. The most serious danger to vision is : **AMU 1986**

A. A blow to the eyeball
B. Fracture through the optic foramen
C. Fracture of cribriform plate
D. Monocular proptosis
E. Horner's syndrome

124. Uniocular Polyopia is seen in which stage of cataract : **AP 1997**

A. Incipient B. Intumescent
C. Mature D. Hypermature

125. Contracted socket occurs because all of the following except : **AP 1988**

A. Chronic low grade infection
B. Chronic mechanical irritation
C. Irradiation
D. Loss of fatty tissue during surgery of enucleation

126. Frill's excision is done in : **AP 1997**

A. Intraocular tumor B. Endophthalmitis
C. Panophthalmitis D. Foreign body in the eye

127. In vicarious menstruation, bleeding may occur from : **Delhi 1982**

A. Nose B. Ear
C. Conjunctiva D. Stomach
E. All of the above

128. Atropine given as antidote in acute physostigmine poisoning shall relieve following symptoms except : **DNB 1989**

A. Circulatory
B. Respiratory
C. Glandular
D. Twitching of skeletal muscles

129. Triad of Still's disease include all except : **Kerala 1997**

A. Episcleritis B. Cataract
C. Band keratopathy D. Uveitis

130. Carotid-cavernous fistula is : **AMC 1983**

A. Associated with a bruit
B. Characterized by exophthalmos
C. The only intracranial traumatic arteriovenous aneurysm
D. All of the above

131. Miners nystagmus is of which type : **UPSC 1985; PGI 1986; JIPMER 1988**

A. Lateral B. Vertical
C. Pendular D. Can be of any type

132. All optical media are clear in : **AMU 1985**

A. Cavernous sinus thrombosis
B. Panophthalmitis
C. Orbital cellulitis
D. None of the above

133. What is Tylosis : **Kerala 1990**

A. Hypertrophy and dropping of eye lid
B. Inversion of eye lid
C. Senile eversion of eye lid
D. Distortion of cilia

134. Ophthalmia nodosa is seen in : **Delhi 1983**

A. Caterpillar hair in the eye
B. Granulomatous uveitis
C. Leprosy
D. Syphilis

135. In Junius-Kuhnt's disease, there is an early disciform degeneration of : **AIIMS 1987**

A. Ciliary body
B. Suspensory ligament of lens
C. Cornea
D. Pigment epithelium
E. None of the above

136. Roth's spots are seen in : **AI 1988**

A. Diabetes mellitus B. S.A.B.E
C. Eale's disease D. Photoretinitis

137. Which of the following is not seen in blunt trauma to eye : **AIIMS 1997**

A. Hyphemia B. Iridiodialysis
C. Retinal haemorrhage D. Double perforation

138. Rubella may present as following except : **AIIMS 1997**

A. Squint B. Leucocoria
C. Trachoma D. Cataract

139. Fuch's fleck is seen in : **DNB 1990**

A. Myopia
B. Hypermetropia
C. Junius-Kuhnt's disease
D. Senile macular degeneration
E. None of the above

140. Fleischer ring is found in : **Delhi 1983**

A. Keratoconus B. Chalcosis
C. Argyrosis D. Buphthalmos
E. None of the above

Ans. **122. C** **123. B** **124. A** **125. D** **126. C** **127. E** **128. D** **129. B** **130. E** **131. C** **132. A** **133. A** **134. A** **135. D** **136. B** **137. D** **138. C** **139. A** **140. A**

141. In patient of AIDS, chorioretinitis is most often caused by : AIIMS 1997
A. Toxoplasma gondii B. Cytomegalo virus
C. Candida D. Herpes simplex

142. Following are seen in ethambutol induced toxic neuritis except : AIIMS 1997
A. Hard exudates B. Impaired colour vision
C. Peripheral field defect D. Central scotoma

143. See saw Nystagmus is seen in : AIIMS 1997
A. Vermis
B. MLF (Medial longitudinal funiculus)
C. Pons
D. Hippocampus

144. Gradual enlargement of optic canal is seen in : AIIMS 1997
A. Retinoblastoma B. Neurofibromatasis
C. Haemangioma D. Meningioma

145. Manifestation of congenital syphilis include all of the following, except : Bihar 1990
A. Extraocular muscle paralysis
B. Chronic dacryocystitis
C. Chorioretinitis
D. Interstitial keratitis

146. Injury to lateral angle of eye causes : Delhi 1984; AIIMS 1985
A. Hyphema B. Lens displacement
C. Vitreous prolapse D. All of the above

147. Most toxic intraocular foreign body is : AIIMS 1985; DNB 1986
A. Glass B. Iron
C. Lead D. Copper

148. Fundal picture characteristic of AIDS is : Rajasthan 1991, 93; DNB 1995
A. Tigroid fundus
B. Owl eye appearance
C. Tomato ketchup appearance
D. Hyperpigmentation of fundus

149. The commonest cause of treatable blindness is : AIIMS 1985
A. Trachoma B. Xerophthalmia
C. Glaucoma D. Injuries

150. In mumps, most common eye lesion is : AIIMS 1997
A. Dacryoadenitis
B. Uveitis
C. Membranous conjunctivitis
D. Chorioretinitis

151. Viral eye infection in adults is commonly caused by : Delhi 1984; AIIMS 1985
A. Herpes B. Adenovirus, strain 8
C. Adenovirus, strain 12 D. Rhinovirus

152. 80 years old man with no history of halos and increased intraocular pressure has : AIIMS 1987
A. Intermittent glaucoma
B. Struge-Weber's syndrome
C. Corneal dystrophy
D. Idiopathic glaucoma

153. Pilocarpine is used in : AIIMS 1986, 87
A. Chronic simple glaucoma
B. Corneal ulcer
C. Secondary glaucoma
D. Acute congestive glaucoma

154. Not a feature of unilateral sympathetic paralysis : AIIMS 1988
A. Mydriasis B. Ptosis
C. Enophthalmos D. Anhydrosis

155. A four years old child presents with white reflex of pupil, proptosis, slight fever, eye pain. The most likely cause is : AIIMS 1988
A. Orbital cellulitis B. Acute frontal sinusitis
C. Retinoblastoma D. Ethmoiditis

156. Exophthalmos is seen in all of the following except : PGI 1985
A. Carotico-cavernous fistula
B. Cavernous sinus thrombosis
C. Internal carotid aneurysm
D. Myaesthenia gravis

157. Corneal nerves are clearly seen in slit lamp examination in : PGI 1985
A. Leprosy B. Tuberculosis
C. Toxocara D. Trachoma

158. Epinephrine is not used in : AIIMS 1997
A. Neovascular glaucoma
B. Aphakic glaucoma
C. Glaucoma with Uveitis
D. Acute Congestive glaucoma

159. Foster Kennedy syndrome is seen in all except : PGI 1987
A. Frontal meningioma
B. Frontal lobe glioma
C. Optic glioma
D. Meningioma of olfactory tract
E. Medulloblastoma in cerebellum

Ans.										
	141. B	142. A	143. A	144. D	145. A	146. D	147. B	148. C	149. B	150. A
	151. B	152. A	153. D	154. A	155. C	156. D	157. A	158. D	159. E	

160. Not true about Pilocarpine use is : **AIIMS 1997**
A. Follicular conjunctivitis
B. Post. synechia
C. Shallow anterior chamber
D. Punctal stenosis

161. Cerebellopontine angle tumor produces following at earliest : **AIIMS 1997**
A. Diplopia
B. Loss of corneal reflex
C. Ipsilateral lateral squint
D. Ipsilateral tongue paralysis

162. Height of lacrimal sac is ——. **AIIMS 1985**
A. 4-6 mm B. 6-8 mm
C. 8-10 mm D. 10-12 mm

163. A 16 years old male comes with injury by a tennis ball. The following can be seen except : **PGI 1983**
A. Hypopyon
B. Hyphema
C. Subluxation of lens
D. Subconjuctival haemorrhage

164. Pulsation unilateral exophathalmus is produced in : **PGI 1986**
A. Post-clinoid aneurysm
B. Carotico caternous fistula
C. Thyrotoxicosis
D. Retinoblastoma

165. Contact lenses may be useful in treatment of all, except : **AIIMS 1981**
A. Keratoconus
B. Refractive anisometropia
C. Fuch's endothelial dystrophy
D. Severe keratoconjunctivitis sicca

166. A 2 months old child has lacrimation in right eye. The following causes constitute differential diagnosis except: **PGI 1985**
A. Congenital dacrocystitis
B. Congenital glaucoma
C. Ophthalmia neonatorum
D. None of the above

167. Retinoma is seen in :
AIIMS 1981; UPSC 1982, 83; AMC 1983, 87
A. Vitamin-A deficiency B. Cataract
C. Injuries D. Uveitis

168. The treatment of maggots in eye is : **Delhi 1990**
A. 10% chloroform B. Cocaine
C. Liquid paraffin D. 10% formalin

169. Following are indications of Botulinum toxin except : **DNB 1997**
A. Osillopsia B. Blepharospasm
C. Indolent corneal ulcer D. Secondary glaucoma
E. Hemifacial synkinesia

170. Intercalary staphyloma occurs at : **AIIMS 1980**
A. Area extending upto 8 mm from limbus
B. Limbus
C. Posterior pole of eye
D. Region of sclera which are perforated by vortex vein
E. Equatorial region

171. The earliest sign of cavernous sinus thrombosis is : **Delhi 1990**
A. Ophthalmoplegia B. Swelling of lids
C. Vomiting D. Proptosis

172. The complications of trabeculectomy are all except : **Delhi 1990**
A. Iritis B. Blockage of wound
C. Choroid detachment D. Retinal detachment

173. Salu's sign is deflection of —— along concealment. **AMU 1986**
A. Retinal vein B. Retinal artery
C. Optic nerve D. Trigeminal nerve

174. Which of the following structure is below 2 mm : **PGI 1994**
A. Insertion of medical rectus
B. Anterior chamber
C. Crystalline lens
D. Optic disc

175. Gaule's spots are related to : **AIIMS 1986**
A. Neurosyphilis
B. Trachoma
C. Neuroparalytic keratitis
D. Diabetes mellitus

176. Botulinum toxin has been successfully used in the following cranial nerve palsies except : **DNB 1997**
A. III B. IV
C. VI D. VII

177. Botulinum toxin-A (light chain) causes dose dependent paralysis by blocking Ca++ dependent release of : **DNB 1996**
A. Sodium B. Acetylcholine
C. Chloride D. Adrenaline

178. Which of the following diseases affect the eye : **PGI 1983, 85**
A. Juvenile rheumatoid artheritis
B. Wilson disease
C. Sjogren's syndrome
D. Leprosy
E. All of the above

Ans.									
160. C	161. B	162. D	163. A	164. B	165. C	166. D	167. A	168. B	169. D
170. B	171. A	172. B	173. A	174. D	175. C	176. D	177. B	178. E	

179. Muscle mostly affected in thyroid ophthalmopathy is : **AIIMS 1982, 85**

A. Lateral rectus B. Inferior rectus
C. Superior rectus D. Medial rectus

180. In unilateral past pointing nystagmus, the site of lesion is : **AI 1989; DNB 1988**

A. Cerebellar hemisphere
B. Lateral semicircular canal
C. Flocculo-nodular lobe
D. Superior semicircular canal

181. In retrobulbar haemorrhage, all are seen except : **Delhi 1988**

A. Limitation of movements
B. Chemosis
C. Proptosis
D. Miosis

182. Blow out fracture of orbit commonly produces : **AP 1993**

A. Deviation of septum
B. Retinal haemorrhage
C. Fracture of nasal bones
D. Fracture of floor of orbit

183. In diabetes mellitus, following lens extraction, all can occur except : **Delhi 1985**

A. Retinal detachment
B. Infection
C. Delayed wound healing
D. Hyphema

184. Early diagnosis of recent perforating injury to eye is by : **Delhi 1985, 88**

A. Chemosis
B. Cyanosis of lids
C. Laceration
D. Decreased intraocular pressure

185. Flourescence angiography may be used to study : **Delhi 1988**

A. Eyelid circulation B. Orbital circulation
C. Retinal vessels D. All of the above

186. Occurrence of cases complaining of diplopia, dysphagia, dysarthria, blurring of vision and muscle weakness could be due to : **Delhi 1984**

A. Diphtheria B. Botulism
C. Infantile beri beri D. Myasthenia gravis

187. The field defect in tobacco amblyopia is : **PGI 1982**

A. Centrocecal B. Central
C. Segmental D. Cecal

188. Following are avascular except : **Delhi 1983**

A. Cornea B. Sclera
C. Vitreous D. Lens

189. A one-month old baby is brought with complaints of photophobia and watering. Clinical examination shows normal tear passages and clear but large cornea. The most likely diagnosis is : **UPSC 1998**

A. Congenital dacryocystitis
B. Interstitial keratitis
C. Keratoconus
D. Buphthalmos

190. A patient with head injury, black eye associated with subconjuctival haemorrhage occurs when there is : **UPSC 1998**

A. Fracture of floor of anterior cranial fossa.
B. Bleeding between the skin and galea aponeurotica.
C. Haemorrhage between galea aponeurotica and pericranium.
D. Fracture of greater wing of sphenoid bone.

191. Acute Stevens-Johnson syndrome can present as : **JIPMER 1998**

A. Anterior uveitis
B. Membranous conjunctivitis
C. Chonioretinitis
D. Vitreous haemorrhage

192. Blindness in Vit.-A deficiency is due to : **JIPMER 1998**

A. Corneal involvement B. Retinopathy
C. Conjunctival scarring D. Uveitis

193. Investigation of choice for endocrine exophthalmos is : **JIPMER 1998**

A. CT B. Orbital ultrasound
C. X-ray D. Tomography

194. Circumference of Globe is ——— mm. **AMU 1987**

A. 25 B. 45
C. 75 D. 85

195. Local steroids are the treatment for : **Delhi 1987**

A. Vernal Catarrh
B. Eale's disease
C. Phylectanular conjuctivitis
D. Trachoma

196. Malignant melanoma of the eye spreads through : **AP 1995**

A. Aqueous humour B. Optic nerve
C. Blood D. Bone

Ans.									
179. B	180. A	181. D	182. D	183. D	184. D	185. D	186. B	187. A	188. B
189. D	190. A	191. B	192. A	193. A	194. C	195. A	196. C		

197. Large Haemangioma of lid and cheek along with glaucoma is seen in : AIIMS 1984, 85

A. Von Recklinghausen's disease
B. Sturge Weber syndrome
C. Von Hippel disease
D. Landau's disease

198. After retrobulbar anaesthesia, pupil responds to : Rajasthan 1990, 94

A. Pilocarpine B. Eserine
C. Both D. None

199. Follicles are not seen in which of the following : AI 1989

A. Spring catarrh
B. Trachoma
C. Adeno virus conjunctivitis
D. Streptococcal conjunctivitis

200. Not a useful form of Vitamin-A : Delhi 1986, 87

A. Retinol B. Retinal
C. Retinoic acid D. None of the above

201. Oculo cardiac reflex is seen during the surgical procedure for : Karnataka 1989

A. Squint B. Cataract
C. Glaucoma D. Dermoid excision

202. Sudden diminition of vision is seen in : Karnataka 1994

A. Eales disease
B. Coats disease
C. Papilloedema
D. Age related macular degeneration

203. Watery secretion from eye is diagnostic of : Delhi 1994

A. Viral Conjunctivitis
B. Vernal catarrh
C. Bacterial conjunctivitis
D. Cataract

204. Mydriasis with fastest action and least duration of cycloplegia is : Delhi 1994; AI 1995

A. Cyclopentolate B. Tropicamide
C. Atropine D. Homatropine

205. A patient complaints of double vision which followed a road traffic accident. Examination shows a slightly sunken left eye with limitation of extra ocular movements. The most likely diagnosis is : UPSC 1994

A. Injury to the lateral rectus muscle
B. Fracture to the pulley of the superior oblique
C. Fracture to orbital floor
D. Orbital haemorrhage

206. A newly married girl of twenty years complains of bilateral loss of vision with no perception of light. Examination of the eye reveals pupil, media and fundus oculi be normal. She is more likely to be suffering from: UPSC 1994

A. Bilateral optic neuritis
B. Pituitary apoplexy
C. Infarction to the occipital lobes
D. Hysterical attack

207. Useful therapy in the treatment of ocular cysticercosis is : UPSC 1994

A. Niclosamide B. Praziquantel
C. Albendazole D. Surgery

208. 5% guanethidine eyedrops are used in : AI 1994

A. Neuroparalytic keratitis
B. Thyrotoxic exophthalmos
C. Horner's syndrome
D. Lid retraction

209. Tubular vision is seen in the following except : AI 1994

A. Chronic simple glaucoma
B. Retinitis pigmentosa
C. High myopia
D. None of the above

210. History of coloured halos is present in all except : MP 1998

A. Mucopurulent conjunctivitis
B. Steroid induced glaucoma
C. Phacogenic glaucoma
D. Closed angle glaucoma

211. The ophthalmic defect commonly seen in patients with Alport syndrome : Bihar 1998

A. Retinitis pigmentosa B. Lenticonus
C. Zonular cataracts D. Optic atrophy

212. Periorbital oedema is not seen in : Kerala 1994, 95

A. Hypothyroidism B. ARF
C. CHF D. Hypopituitarism

213. The following are regarded as being important causes of ocular infection in AIDS patients : AIIMS 1986

A. Histoplasmosis B. Mycobacterium avium
C. Cryptococcus D. Toxoplasmosis
E. Herpes zoster

214. True about Neodymium-YAG laser except : DNB 1989

A. Photocoagulates
B. Vaporizes
C. Forms a plasma
D. Is not visible
E. Creates mechanical waves

Ans.	197. B	198. C	199. A	200. C	201. B	202. A	203. A	204. B	205. B	206. D
	207. D	208. B	209. C	210. B	211. B	212. D	213. D	214. A		

215. False about Stargardt's disease : AIIMS 1983, 86
A. Is inherited.
B. Presents in the third or fourth decade.
C. Characteristically displays an abnormal ERG.
D. May exhibit a 'dark choroid' on fluorescein angiography.
E. Is a cause of 'bull's eye' macular changes

216. Proptosis may be pulsatile when caused by all except : AIIMS 1986
A. Arteriovenous malformations
B. Rhabdomyosarcoma
C. Meningoencephalocele
D. Frontal mucocele
E. Neurofibromatosis

217. Features of Stickler's syndrome include all except : AIIMS 1985
A. Autosomal dominant inheritance
B. Micrognathia
C. Glaucoma
D. Marfanoid habitus
E. Mitral regurgitation

218. The 'cherry-red spot at the macula' syndromes include all except : AIIMS 1985
A. Weil-Marchesani syndrome
B. Tay-Sachs syndrome
C. Sandhoff's disease
D. Niemann Pick disease
E. Sialidosis

219. The following syndromes involving the eye may have associated renal abnormalities except : PGI 1986
A. Alport's syndrome
B. Aniridia
C. Ehlers-Danlos syndrome
D. Lowe's syndrome
E. Leber's congenital amaurosis

220. The following are features of Mobius' syndrome except : DNB 1989
A. Skeletal abnormalities
B. Facial nerve palsy
C. Abduction weakness
D. Autosomal dominant inheritance
E. Hypoplasia of the tongue

221. Useful tests and investigations in the diagnosis of sarcoidosis includes all except : AIIMS 1984
A. HLA B27 states B. Transbronchial biopsy
C. Urine calcium D. Mantoux test
E. Chest X-rays

222. The pain in Tolosa Hunt syndrome is best treated with : DNB 1998
A. Atropine B. Corticosteroids
C. Aspirin D. Ciprofloxacin

223. Hard contact lens is most useful in : Karnataka 1994
A. Arresting myopia B. Correcting astigmatism
C. Drug delivery D. Keratoconus

224. Enucleation in the donor eye should be performed within —— hours of death. Karnataka 1994
A. 2 B. 6
C. 24 D. 48

225. Shortest acting mydriatic among following is : AI 1995
A. Homatropine B. Cyclopentolate
C. Atropine D. Hyoscine

226. Ocular manifestation of Sturge Weber syndrome is : Kerala 1994
A. Hemangioma of choroid and glaucoma
B. Leisch nodules
C. Pulsating exophthalmos
D. Retinal haemorrhage

227. Adenovirus causes : Kerala 1994
A. Keratoconjunctivitis B. Diarrhoea
C. Parotid enlargement D. Lymphoma

228. Intraocular lens implantation is done best in following except : PGI 1993
A. Ciliary groove
B. Iris support
C. In the lag
D. Angle of anterior chamber

229. Bare orbit is seen in all except : PGI 1994, 97
A. Meningioma B. Enucleation of the eye
C. Metastasis D. Phthisis

230. Cycloplegic drugs are following except : PGI 1994
A. Tropicamide B. Cyclopentolate
C. Homatropine D. Pilocarpine

231. Ocular absorption of a drug is increased by : PGI 1994
A. Strong alkali base B. Strong acidic base
C. Weak Acid base D. None of the above

232. In DM, floaters indicate : Delhi 1995
A. Post. vitreous haemorrhage
B. Retinal tear
C. Proliferative RP
D. Neovascularization

Ans.										
	215. B	216. A	217. E	218. A	219. C	220. D	221. A	222. B	223. D	224. B
	225. A	226. A	227. A	228. A	229. A	230. D	231. A	232. A		

233. Superficial layer of tear film is formed by : PGI 1995

A. Sclera B. Air
C. Lacrimal gland D. Cornea

234. Index of refraction of PMMA lens is : DNB 1995

A. 1.17 B. 1.26
C. 1.49 D. 1.57

235. Flashing of light is an earliest sign of : UPSC 1994; Rohtak 1996

A. Cataract B. Glaucoma
C. Retinal detachment D. Corneal opacity

236. Berlin's oedema is seen in : PGI 1996, AIIMS 1983, 89, 96

A. Thermal injury B. Radiation
C. Concussion injury D. Penetration injury

237. Which of the following causes deposition of melanin pigment in Descemet membrane : PGI 1996

A. Chloroquine B. Penicillamine
C. Phenothiazine D. Paracetamol

238. Most common ocular finding in AIDS is : PGI 1996

A. Corneal dystrophy B. Cottonwool spots
C. Retinal detachment D. Glaucoma

239. Choreoretinitis in AIDS is caused by : PGI 1996

A. EBV B. Toxoplasmosis
C. Herpes D. Adenovirus

240. The carotico-cavernous fistula is best treated by : AI 1997

A. Embolisation
B. Evisceration
C. Internal carotid artery ligation
D. No specific treatment

241. The weakest wall of the human Orbit is : Orissa 1998

A. Roof B. Medial wall
C. Floor D. Lateral wall

242. A patient presented with pain and circumcorneal congestion of the right eye. On examination, the right pupil is constricted. The anterior chamber is of normal depth. The anterior chamber of the left eye is shallow. Which of the following could be the diagnosis : AIIMS 1999

A. Glaucoma B. Uveitis
C. Retinal detachment D. Trachoma

243. A person sustained blunt trauma to the right eye with immediate loss of vision. On examination the anterior chamber of the eye is deep. The cause could be : AIIMS 1999

A. Hyphema B. Dislocation of lens
C. Retinal detachment D. Iridodialysis

244. In non-proliferation diabetes, most common cause of blindness: AIIMS 1999

A. Sub retinal Haemorrhage
B. Macular edema
C. Retinal detachment
D. Vitreous haemorrhage

245. The most accepted modality of treatment of -2D myopia in a 13 years old girl is : UPSC 2005

A. Spectacles B. Excimer laser
C. Contact lens D. Radial keratotomy

246. Aniseikonia refers to : PGI 1999

A. Difference in the corneal diameter
B. Difference in the image size (retinal image)
C. Difference in the refractive power
D. Difference in image colour

247. Which is not a part of the pupillary reflex : PGI 1999

A. Lateral geniculate body
B. Pre-tectal area
C. Retina
D. Edinger-Westiphal nucleus

248. Yag laser is used in treatment of : PGI 1999

A. Pterygium B. After cataract
C. Retinal detachment D. Retinitis

249. Axial proptosis is seen in: JIPMER 2000

A. Optic nerve glioma
B. Blow out fracture of orbit
C. Tumour pressing from manillary antrum
D. Frontal mucocele

250. Size of incision given for phacoemulsification is : Delhi 2001

A. 1-2 mm B. 3-5 mm
C. 5-8 mm D. 8-10 mm

251. Safe and effective method of sterilization of surgical eye instruments is : Delhi 2001

A. Acetone B. Formaline
C. Autoclaving D. Boiling

252. Most common cause of post-operative endophthalmitis following cataract surgery is : Delhi 2001

A. Viral B. Bacterial
C. Fungal D. Parasitic

253. Blunt injury to the eye often causes all except : DNB 2001

A. Angle recession B. Anterior polar cataract
C. Berlin edema D. Avulsion of optic nerve

254. Which of the following is not an inert foreign body: MAHE 2001

A. Aluminium B. Silver
C. Gold D. Platinum

Ans.										
	233. C	234. C	235. C	236. C	237. A	238. B	239. B	240. C	241. B	242. A
	243. B	244. B	245. B	246. B	247. A	248. B	249. D	250. B	251. C	252. B
	253. D	254. A								

255. **Fixed dilated pupil is seen in : MAHE 2001**
A. Oculomotor palsy B. Trochlear palsy
C. Abducens palsy D. None

256. **In panophthalmitis, the treatment of choice is : MAHE 2001**
A. Enucleation B. Evisceration
C. Exanteration D. None

257. **The best diagnosis for Best disease is : JIPMER 2002**
A. EOG B. EEG
C. ERG D. ENG

258. **Which of the following acts on the uveoscleral tract : SGPGI 2002**
A. Levobunol B. Epinephrine
C. Lanatoprost D. Timolol maleate

259. **A patient presented with unilateral ptosis and diplopia and on examination was found to have decreased movement of eyeball in all directions. The patient also complains of difficulty in reading newsprint. The diagnosis is : SGPGI 2002**
A. Myasthenia gravis B. Oculomotor palsy
C. Trochlear palsy D. Facial nerve palsy

260. **Night blindness is caused by all except : SGPGI 2002**
A. Retinitis pigmentosa
B. Cone dystrophy
C. Xeroderma pigmentosa
D. Chronic Tobacco use

261. **In a patient with color blindness all the following are true except : SGPGI 2002**
A. It is misnomer as it is actually a color defect and not blindness.
B. There is normal visual acuity.
C. Most common anomaly is blue green defect.
D. More common in males.

262. **Cone is the most sensitive cell in the retina. It picks up images from a mix of red, blue and green colors. Abnormality in color perception needing increased use of red color for normal perception is : AI 2002**
A. Protanomaly B. Deuteranomaly
C. Tritanomaly D. Malingerer

263. **Pink-fundus is seen in : Maharashtra 2000**
A. Papilloedema B. Pseudo-papilloedema
C. Papillitis D. Retinitis pigmentosa

264. **Meiosis + anhidrosis + ptosis : CMC 2001**
A. Horner's syndrome
B. Marfan's syndrome
C. Millard-Gubler syndrome
D. All of the above

265. **Chalcosis bulbi is related to : A.P. 2002**
A. Coal B. Copper
C. Iron D. Gold

266. **Frill excision is done in : BHU-2002**
A. Endophthalmitis
B. Panophthalmitis
C. Foreign body in the eye
D. Cataract

267. **Which one of the following is the serious complication of degenerative myopia in the eye : UPSC 2002**
A. Retinal detachment
B. Vitreous liquifaction
C. Myopic crescent
D. Posterior staphyloma

268. **Which one of the following conditions does not cause Pseudoexophthalmos : UPSC 2002**
A. High myopia
B. Lid retraction
C. Optic nerve glioma
D. Facial nerve paralysis

269. **A one-year-old child having leucocoria was detected to be having a unilateral, large retinoblastoma filling half the globe. Current therapy would involve : AIIMS 2002**
A. Enucleation
B. Chemotherapy followed by local dyes.
C. Direct Laser ablation using photo dynamic cryotherapy.
D. Scleral radiotherapy followed by chemotherapy.

270. **A 2-years-old child presented with leucocoria in the right eye since 2 months. On examination, a total retinal detachment was present in the same eye. Ultrasound B scan revealed a heterogenous subretinal mass with calcification, associated with a retinal detachment. The most likely clinical diagnosis is : AIIMS 2002**
A. Coats disease B. Retinoblastoma
C. Toxocariasis D. Retinal tuberculoma

271. **While working in the neonatal ICU, your team delivers a premature infant at 27 weeks of gestation and weighing 1500 gms. How soon will you request fundus examination by an ophthalmologist : AIIMS 2002**
A. Immediately
B. 3-4 weeks after delivery
C. At 34 weeks gestational age
D. At 40 weeks gestational age

Ans. 255. A 256. B 257. A 258. C 259. B 260. B 261. C 262. A 263. B 264. A
265. B 266. B 267. A 268. C 269. A 270. B 271. B

272. A friend of yours has a spectacle correction of - 6.0 and 8.0. He telephones you one morning and tells that he has started seeing some opacities floating in from his eye and that his vision has decreased slightly over the last few days. As an intern in the ophthalmology section, what would you do : AIIMS 2002

A. Reassure
B. Refraction and prescribe a new spectacle
C. Direct ophthalmoscopy
D. Indirect ophthalmoscopy

273. A 17 years old girl with keratitis and severe pain in the eye came to the hospital and Acanthomoeba keratitis was suspected. The patient gave the history of following four points. Out of these which is not a risk factor for Acanthomoeba keratitis : AIIMS 2002

A. Extended wear contact lens
B. Exposure to dirty water
C. Corneal trauma
D. Squamous blepharitis

274. Haab's striae are seen in : CUPGME-2002

A. Acute angle closure glaucoma
B. Open angle glaucoma
C. Buphthalmos
D. Retinoblastoma

275. Phakoemulsification with I.O.L is done in : CUPGME-2002

A. Anterior chamber B. Posterior chamber
C. In the capsular bag D. In the plane of iris

276. A vitreous aspirate has been collected in an emergency at 9 pm. What advice you like to give to the staff on duty regarding the overnight storage of the sample : AI 2003

A. The sample should be kept at 4 Degrees C.
B. The sample should be incubated at 37 Degrees C.
C. The sample should be refrigerated in deep freezer.
D. The sample should be refrigerated for the initial 3 hours and then incubated at 37 Degrees C.

277. A 1 yr old child having leucocoria was detected to be having a unilateral, large retinoblastoma filling half the globe. Current therapy would involve : AI 2003

A. Enucleation
B. Chemotherapy with local dyes
C. Direct Laser Ablation using photodynamic cryotherapy
D. Scleral radiotherapy followed by chemotherapy

278. A patient is on follow-up with you after enucleation of a painful blind eye. After enucleation of the eyeball, a proper sized artificial prosthetic eye is advised after a post-operative period of : AI 2003

A. About 10 days B. About 20 days
C. 6-8 weeks D. 12-24 weeks

279. A lady wants LASIK surgery for her daughter. She asks for your opinion. All of the following things are suitable for performing LASIK except : AI 2003

A. Myopia of 4D
B. Age of 15 years
C. Stable refraction for 1 year
D. Corneal thickness of 600 microns

280. Vortex vein invasion is commonly seen in : AI 2003

A. Retinoblastoma B. Malignant melanoma
C. Optic nerve glioma D. Medullo-epitheliomas

281. Laser iridotomy is done for : JIPMER 2003

A. Buphthalmos
B. Primary angle closure glaucoma
C. Staphyloma
D. After cataract

282. Scleromalacia perforans is seen in : JIPMER 2003

A. Rheumatoid arthritis B. Sicca syndromes
C. Vitamin-A deficiency D. Herpetic keratitis

283. Photopsia is seen in : JIPMER 2003

A. Optic neuritis
B. Retinal detachment
C. Open angle of Glaucoma
D. Myopia

284. Frequent changes in glasses is associated with which of the following diseases : MAHE 2003

A. Closed angle glaucoma
B. Open angle glaucoma
C. Senile cataract
D. Vitreous haeamorrhage

285. Increased field of vision is associated with which of the following : MAHE 2003

A. Yellow B. Blue
C. White D. Green

286. Arlt's line is seen in : AI 2004

A. Vernal keratoconjunctivitis
B. Pterygium
C. Ocular pemphigoid
D. Trachoma

Ans.									
272. D	273. D	274. C	275. C	276. A	277. A	278. C	279. B	280. A	281. A
282. A	283. A	284. B	285. A	286. D					

287. **A 10-months-old child weighing 8 kg has Bitot spots in both eyes. Which of the following is the most appropriate schedule to prescribe vitamin-A to this child:** **AI 2004**

A. 2 lack units intramuscular (IM) day 0, 14
B. 1 lack units IM on day 0, 14
C. 2 lack units IM on day 0, 1 and 14
D. 1 lack units IM on day 0, 1 and 14

288. **All of the following can cause a white pupillary reflex except:** **AI 2004**

A. Retinoblastoma B. Cataract
C. Retrolental fibroplasia D. Glaucoma

289. **A 12 years old girl with tremors and emotional lability has a golden brown discoloration of Descement's membrane. The most likely diagnosis is:** **AI 2004**

A. Fabry's disease
B. Wilson disease
C. Glycogen storage disease
D. Acute rheumatic fever

290. **Latanoprost used topically in glaucoma primarily acts by:** **AI 2004**

A. Decreasing aqueous humor formation
B. Increasing uveoscleral outflow
C. Releasing pupillary block
D. Increasing trabecular outflow

291. **The most common condition of inherited blindness due to mitochondrial chromosomal anomaly is:** **AI 2004**

A. Retinopathy of prematurity
B. Leber's hereditary optic neuropathy
C. Retinitis pigmentosa
D. Retinal detachment

292. **"Photo dynamic therapy" is used in the eye for the following disease:** **AI 2004**

A. Cataract
B. Glaucoma
C. Uveitis
D. Wet AMD (age related macular degeneration)

293. **All are ocular emergencies except:** **AI 2004**

A. Angle closure glaucoma
B. Central serous retinopathy
C. Retinal detachment
D. Central retinal arterial occulsion

294. **A two months old child presents with epiphora and regurgitation. The most probable diagnosis is:** **AI 2004**

A. Mucopurulent conjunctivitis
B. Buphthalmos
C. Congenital dacryocystitis
D. Encysted mucocele

295. **Which prominent ocular manifestation is associated with Marfan's syndrome:** **AI 2004**

A. Microcornea B. Microspherophakia
C. Megalocornea D. Ectopia lentis

296. **"Angry sun appearance" in fundoscopy is a feature of:** **Karnataka 2005**

A. Primary optic atrophy B. Papilloedema
C. Pappilitis D. Drusen's rings

297. **The mother of a one and half year old child gives history of a white reflex from one eye for the past 1 month. On computed tomography scan of the orbit there is calcification seen within the globe. The most likely diagnosis is:** **AI 2005**

A. Congenital cataract B. Retinoblastoma
C. Endophthalmitis D. Coats disease

298. **A 25 years old male gives history of sudden painless loss of vision in one eye for the past 2 weeks. There is no history of trauma. On examination the anterior segment is normal but there is no fundal glow. Which one of the following is the most likely cause:** **AI 2005**

A. Vitreous haemorrhage
B. Optic atrophy
C. Development cataract
D. Acute attack of angle closure glaucoma

299. **Horner's syndrome is characterized by all of the following except:** **AI 2005**

A. Miosis B. Enophthalmos
C. Ptosis D. Cycloplegia

300. **Under the WHO 'Vision 2020' programme, the SAFE strategy is adopted for which of the following diseases:** **AI 2005**

A. Trachoma B. Glaucoma
C. Diabetic retinopathy D. Onchocerciasis

301. **An 18 years old boy comes to the eye casualty with history of injury with a tennis ball. On examination there is no perforation but there is hyphaema. The most likely source of the blood is:** **AI 2005**

A. Iris vessels
B. Circulus iridis major
C. Circulus iridis minor
D. Short posterior ciliary vessels

302. **Which one of the following drugs does not affect accommodation:** **UPSC 2005**

A. Pilocarpine B. Atropine
C. Physostigmine D. Dopamine

Ans.									
287. D	288. D	289. B	290. B	291. B	292. D	293. B	294. C	295. D	296. B
297. B	298. A	299. D	300. A	301. B	302. D				

303. **In fetus Angio genesis in eye involve all except :** AI 2009

A. TNF b
B. IL-8
C. BFGF
D. VEGF

304. **All are true about Lambert Eaton syndrome except :** AI 2009

A. Spares ocular muscle
B. Tensilon test positive
C. Proximal muscle involvement
D. Repeat nerve stimulation improve muscle strength

305. **A patient with clinically significant diabetic macular edema and non-progressive diabetic retinopathty was treated with Macular grid photocoagulation. The patient still has vitreomacular traction. What is the preferred treatment :** AIIMS 2011

A. Intravitreal bevacizumab
B. Pars plana vitrectomy
C. Repeat macular grid photocoagulation
D. Augmented macula photocoagulation

306. **Baby born prematurely at 29 wks. On examination at 42 wks with ROP, both eyes shows stage 2 zone 1 plus disease how will you manage the patient :** AIIMS 2011

A. Examine the patient after 1 week
B. Laser photocoagulation of both eyes
C. Laser photocoagulation of worse eye, follow up of other eye
D. Vitreoretinal surgery

307. **A 25 years old lady presents with sudden, severe bilateral loss of vision more so on right side with no perception of light. Rest of the examination including pupillary reflex, fundus & optokinetic nystagmus are normal. She was able to touch tips of her finger with right eye closed but not with left eye closed. most likely diagnosis :** AIIMS 2011

A. Optic neuritis
B. Anterior ischaemic optic neuropathy
C. CMV retinitis
D. Functional visual loss

308. **Dilator pupillae is supplied by :** AIIMS 2011

A. Post ganglionic parasympathetic fibres from Edinger Westphal nucleus
B. Post ganglionic sympathetic fibres from cervical sympathetic chain
C. III nerve
D. Sympathetic fibres from frontoorbital branch of V nerve

309. **Mizuo phenomenon is seen in :AIIMS 2011**

A. Fundus albipathicus B. Fundus flavimaculatus
C. Oguchi's disease D. Choroideremia

310. **Topical administration of 1% pilocarpine failed to produce pupillary constriction in a patient who had a large dilated pupil. What could be most probable reason :** AIIMS 2011

A. Diabetic III cranial nerve palsy
B. Adie's tonic pupil
C. Pharmacological blockade
D. Uncal herniation

311. **Methanol causes blindenss by causing damage to :** DNB 2011

A. Nerve cells B. Ganglion cells
C. Lens D. Choroid

312. **Alkali injury causing global penetration can result in :** DNB 2011

A. Symblepharon B. Optic neuritis
C. Retinal detachment D. Cataract

313. **Eales disease is characterized by following except :** DNB 2011

A. Recurrent retinal haemorrhage
B. Recurrent vitreous haemorrhage
C. Neovascularization
D. Preliferative retinopathy

314. **Shortest acting mydriatic is :** DNB 2011

A. Tropicamide B. Cyclopentolate
C. Oxyphenium D. Hyosine

315. **Second most common malignancy is a patient with retinoblastoma :** DNB 2011

A. Nephroblastoma B. Osteosarcoma
C. Neuroblastoma D. Craniopharyngiona

316. **Posterior staphyloma is associated with :** DNB 2011

A. Pathological myopia
B. Retinoblastoma
C. Acid injury
D. Sympathetic ophthalmia

317. **Laser used for iridotomy :** DNB 2011

A. Nd-Yag laser B. Argon
C. Helium-Neon D. Krypton

318. **Sudden painless loss of vision is seen in all, except :** DNB 2011

A. Papilloedema B. Amblyopia
C. Vitreous haemorrhage D. CRVO

319. **Chronic steroid use causes :** DNB 2011

A. Open angle glaucoma
B. Conjunctival papillomatosis
C. Uveitis
D. Cataract

320. **A traveller with foreign body sensation in eyes and swelling of joints, the cause is :** DNB 2011

A. Reiter's disease B. Behcet's disease
C. Eales disease D. Syphilis

Ans.									
303. B	304. A	305. B	306. B	307. D	308. B	309. C	310. C	311. A	312. A
313. D	314. A	315. B	316. A	317. A	318. A	319. A	320. A		

321. **Retinoids ard vitamin A decrease incidence of which cancer of :** DNB 2011
A. Bladder B. Cervix
C. Stomach D. Liver

322. **Not a cause of night blindness :** DNB 2011
A. Vitamin A deficiency
B. High myopia
C. Eales disease
D. None of the above

323. **Dalen Fuch's nodular are seen in :** DNB 2011
A. Eales disease
B. Allergic conjunctivitis
C. Sympathetic ophthalmia
D. Retinal detachment

324. **Not a cause of visual loss in hypertension :** DNB 2011
A. Vitreous haemorrhage
B. Glaucoma
C. Cotton wool spots
D. Retinal detachment

325. **Schirmer's test is for which nerve :** DNB 2011
A. V B. VII
C. IX D. X

326. **In India vision 2020 includes following except :** AI 2012
A. Cataract
B. Refractive errors
C. Vitamin A deficiency
D. Diabetic retinopathy

327. **A 20 year old with night blindness and tunnel vision has :** AI 2012
A. Optic atrophy
B. Pigmendary retinal dystrophy
C. Acute congestive glaucoma
D. Neurosyphilis

328. **CRAO is seen in :** AI 2012
A. DM
B. CMV retinitis
C. Orbital mucormycos
D. Steven Johnson syndrome

Ans. 321. B 322. B 323. C 324. B 325. B 326. C 327. B 328. A

EXPLANATIONS OF MISCELLANEOUS

1. Ans. — C. After cataract
2. Ans. — B. Open angle glaucoma
3. Ans. — A. Iridocyclitis

   There is severe pain in the eye in association with ciliary congestion, muddy colour of iris with small, irregular sluggish pupil and presence of K.P.
4. Ans. — C. Malignant glaucoma
5. Ans. — C. Cystic blebs of iris
6. Ans. — A. Myopia

   Hypermetropia occurs when blood sugar falls and myopia when blood sugar rises.
7. Ans. — A. Glaucoma
8. Ans. — A. Keratoconus
9. Ans. — B. Glaucoma
10. Ans. — D. Herpes zoster
11. Ans. — A. Interstitial keratitis
12. Ans. — A. Complicated cataract

    Appearance of iridescent coloured particles called Polychromatic lustre of reds, greens and blues are seen. Cataract is 'bread crumb' type.
13. Ans. — A. Keratoconus
14. Ans. — A. Cataract
15. Ans. — A. Prostigmine

    In myasthenia gravis, there is ptosis and defect in eye movements due to weakness of muscles. It improves with cholinergic drugs.
16. Ans. — C. Carotid artery occlusion
17. Ans. — A. Near limbus
18. Ans. — C. Night blindness

    Night blindness is earliest symptom and conjunctival xerosis is earliest sign.
19. Ans. — D. Retinoblastoma
20. Ans. — B. Folliculosis
21. Ans. — D. Toxocariasis
22. Ans. — B. Hepatolenticular degeneration
23. Ans. — C. Thyrotoxicosis
24. Ans. — C. Superior quadrantic field defect
25. Ans. — D. Resection of the levator
26. Ans. — E. All of the above

    Angioid streaks are dark brown or pigmented streaks which anastomose with each other and may be mistaken for blood vessels. They are due to changes in elastic tissue of Bruch's membrane. The causes are pseudoxanthoma elasticum, Paget's disease of bone, Ehlers- Danlos syndrome dysbetali-poproteinemia and sickle cell disease.
27. Ans. — E. All of the above
28. Ans. — E. All of the above
29. Ans. — E. All of the above
30. Ans. — C. Uveal tract
31. Ans. — E. 30 cc
32. Ans. — E. Abducens nerve
33. Ans. — B. 8
34. Ans. — C. Temporal cortex
35. Ans. — A. Post. opacities
36. Ans. — B. Descemet's membrane

    Schalbe's line is prominent end of Descemet's membrane of cornea.
37. Ans. — C. Third cranial nerve
38. Ans. — B. Long suture
39. Ans. — A. Vitreous haemorrhage
40. Ans. — C. Ectopic of the pupil
41. Ans. — A. Autosomal recessive inheritance
42. Ans. — D. Epibulbar dermoids
43. Ans. — B. The congenital form usually present at the age of 5 or under.

44. Ans. — A. Echinococcus granulosus

45. Ans. — B. Irrigation with saline

For photophthalmia, cold compress, a drop of xylocaine, 4% atropine and steroid drops with pad and bandage relieve the symptoms.

46. Ans. — D. All of the above

47. Ans. — C. Descemet's membrane

48. Ans. — C. Copper

49. Ans. — D. Ciliary processes are abnormal

50. Ans. — D. Exposure keratopathy

51. Ans. — C. The PA view shows the sac to be continuous with the nasolacrimal duct.

52. Ans. — C. 7.5

53. Ans. — E. None of the above

54. Ans. — C. Retinoblastoma

55. Ans. — B. Muller's muscle

56. Ans. — E. All of the above

57. Ans. — A. Cataract

58. Ans. — D. Tropicamide

It is used in 0.5-2% concentration, has onset of cycloplegia for 20-25 min and duration is 6 hours.

59. Ans. — A. Cycrimine

60. Ans. — B. Posterolateral, Post-cerebral

61. Ans. — D. Convergence does not commence before 2 months.

62. Ans. — B. Ant. Capsule of lens

It is seen in ant. lens capsule.

63. Ans. — B. Retrobulbar neuritis

Lack of sustained constriction of the pupil to light, if it can be placed beyond dispute, is of greatest diagnostic significance.

64. Ans. — E. Pre-operative narrow angle

65. Ans. — D. Scheie's operation

66. Ans. — C. Iridencleisis

67. Ans. — B. Trephine

68. Ans. — A. Cyclodialysis

69. Ans. — E. Nasopharyngeal carcinoma

70. Ans. — E. Rupture of a supraclinoid aneurysm

71. Ans. — A. Reaction due to copper of foreign body in the cornea.

72. Ans. — B. Retinoblastoma

73. Ans. — B. Epicanthus

74. Ans. — C. I (iii) II (iv) III (ii) IV (v) V (i)

75. Ans. — A. Ant. chamber

76. Ans. — A. Vitreous haemorrhage

77. Ans. — A. Cornea

78. Ans. — D. Limbus.

79. Ans. — C. Cavernous sinus thrombosis

80. Ans. — C. Optic Disc

81. Ans. — D. Nicotinic acid deficiency

82. Ans. — B. In keratomileusis removal of convex lens from the corneal disc will make the eye more hypermetropic.

83. Ans. — A. Lipid material

84. Ans. — C. Macula

85. Ans. — C. Lens extraction

86. Ans. — C. Copper compound

It is seen in Wilson's disease.

87. Ans. — E. All of the above

88. Ans. — A. Retinal detachment

89. Ans. — D. Herpes zoster

90. Ans. — B. Esotropia

91. Ans. — D. Being incapable of metastasizing

92. Ans. — C. Ciliary epithelium

93. Ans. — B. Endothelial changes most marked in periphery

94. Ans. — B. Panophthalmitis

95. Ans. — C. Measles

96. Ans. — A. Diabetes mellitus

97. Ans. — B. Choroid

Malignant melanoma is most common primary intraocular tumour of adults seen in 40-70 years of age. It arises from neural chest derived pigment cells of uvea as a solitary tumor and is usually unilateral. Callender classifies it into six types (Spindle-A, Spindle-B, fascicular, Epitheloid cell, Mixed cell and necrotic type).

98. Ans. — B. Meningioma

99. Ans. — D. All of the above

100. Ans. — A. Weber's syndrome

101. Ans. — C. Cholesterol crystals

102. Ans. — A. Episcleritis

103. Ans. — C. Ultra-violet rays

104. Ans. — C. 8-9 mm behind the limbus

105. Ans. — E. All of the above

106. Ans. — B. They are situated at a superficial level than the retinal vessels.

107. Ans. — B. Upper part

108. Ans. — E. None of the above

The condition in which the oscillations are very large and easily seen and are to a great extent independent of the light falling upon the eye. This is called hippus. It depends on the rhythmic acitivity of the nervous centres and is not a peripheral phenomenon. It is found in association with multiple sclerosis.

109. Ans. — C. Pupil does not react to light

110. Ans. — C. I (v) II (iv) III (i) IV (iii) V (ii)

111. Ans. — D. Ectropion

112. Ans. — A. Macula

Retina is most often affected (i.e. burnt).

113. Ans. — E. All of the above

114. Ans. — D. Sphenoid wing meningioma

115. Ans. — E. All of the above

116. Ans. — D. None of the above

117. Ans. — C. Astigmatism

118. Ans. — A. Panophthalmitis

119. Ans. — D. Absolute glaucoma

120. Ans. — C. Juvenile xanthogranuloma

121. Ans. — A. In the treatment of retinoblastoma, seeds 6 mm diameter.

122. Ans. — C. Blood staining of cornea

123. Ans. — B. Fracture through the optic foramen

124. Ans. — A. Incipient

125. Ans. — D. Loss of fatty tissue during surgery of enucleation

126. Ans. — C. Panophthalmitis

127. Ans. — E. All of the above

128. Ans. — D. Twitching of skeletal muscles

129. Ans. — B. Cataract

130. Ans. — E. All of the above

131. Ans. — C. Pendular

Miner's nystagmus is an occupational disease confined to workers of coal mine. Lack of illumination is cause. Nystagmus is pendular which may be horizontal, vertical or rotatory.

132. Ans. — A. Cavernous sinus thrombosis

133. Ans. — A. Hypertrophy and dropping of eye lid

134. Ans. — A. Caterpillar hair in the eye

135. Ans. — D. Pigment epithelium

136. Ans. — B. S.A.B.E

137. Ans. — D. Double perforation

138. Ans. — C. Trachoma

139. Ans. — A. Myopia

140. Ans. — A. Keratoconus

Fleischer ring is seen at base of cone in keratoconus on slit lamp examination.

141. Ans. — B. Cytomegalo virus

142. Ans. — A. Hard exudates

143. Ans. — A. Vermis

144. Ans. — D. Meningioma

145. Ans. — A. Extraocular muscle paralysis

146. Ans. — D. All of the above

147. Ans. — B. Iron

Common foreign bodies are chips of iron and steel (90%) particles of glass, stone, lead pellets, copper percussion caps, aluminium, plastic and wood. Siderosis bulbi (due to iron) occur after 2 months to 2 years of injury. Earliest changes are reported after 9 days of trauma.

148. Ans. — C. Tomato ketchup appearance

149. Ans. — B. Xerophthalmia

Vitamin-A deficiency is one of the commonest cause of treatable blindness.

150. Ans. — A. Dacryoadenitis

151. Ans. — B. Adenovirus, strain 8

152. Ans. — A. Intermittent glaucoma

153. Ans. — D. Acute congestive glaucoma

154. Ans. — A. Mydriasis

155. Ans. — C. Retinoblastoma

156. Ans. — D. Myaesthenia gravis

157. Ans. — A. Leprosy

158. Ans. — D. Acute Congestive glaucoma

159. Ans. — E. Medulloblastoma in cerebellum

There is optic atrophy in one eye and papilloedema in other.

160. Ans. — C. Shallow anterior chamber

161. Ans. — B. Loss of corneal reflex

162. Ans. — D. 10-12 mm

Lacrimal sac is 15 mm in length and 5-6 mm in breadth. Nasolacrimal duct is 15-18 mm long.

163. Ans. — A. Hypopyon
164. Ans. — B. Carotico caternous fistula
165. Ans. — C. Fuch's endothelial dystrophy
166. Ans. — D. None of the above
167. Ans. — A. Vitamin-A deficiency
168. Ans. — B. Cocaine
169. Ans. — D. Secondary glaucoma
170. Ans. — B. Limbus
171. Ans. — A. Ophthalmoplegia
172. Ans. — B. Blockage of wound
173. Ans. — A. Retinal vein

Deflection of veins at AV crossings in hypertensive retinopathy is called Salu's sign .

174. Ans. — D. Optic disc
175. Ans. — C. Neuroparalytic keratitis
176. Ans. — D. VII
177. Ans. — B. Acetylcholine
178. Ans. — E. All of the above
179. Ans. — B. Inferior rectus
180. Ans. — A. Cerebellar hemisphere
181. Ans. — D. Miosis
182. Ans. — D. Fracture of floor of orbit
183. Ans. — D. Hyphema
184. Ans. — D. Decreased intraocular pressure
185. Ans. — D. All of the above
186. Ans. — B. Botulism
187. Ans. — A. Centrocecal

Tabacco amblyopia occurs in men who are generally pipe smokers, heavy drinkers and have a diet deficient in proteins and Vitamin B-complex and hence also called tabacco-alcohol amblyopia. There is bilateral progressive impair-ment in central vision. There are bilateral centrocecal scotomas with diffuse margins which are not easily defined. Disc is normal or has slight temporal pallor.

188. Ans. — B. Sclera
189. Ans. — D. Buphthalmos
190. Ans. — A. Fracture of floor of anterior cranial fossa
191. Ans. — B. Membranous conjunctivitis
192. Ans. — A. Corneal involvement

Initially there is corneal xerosis followed by ulceration and keratomalacia.

193. Ans. — A. CT
194. Ans. — C. 75
195. Ans. — A. Vernal Catarrh
196. Ans. — C. Blood
197. Ans. — B. Sturge Weber syndrome
198. Ans. — C. Both
199. Ans. — A. Spring catarrh

In spring catarrh, hard, flat papillae are seen separated by furrows giving a cobblestone appearance (over upper palpebral conjunctiva).

200. Ans. — C. Retinoic acid
201. Ans. — B. Cataract
202. Ans. — A. Eales disease
203. Ans. — A. Viral Conjunctivitis
204. Ans. — B. Tropicamide
205. Ans. — B. Fracture to the pulley of the superior oblique.
206. Ans. — D. Hysterical attack
207. Ans. — D. Surgery
208. Ans. — B. Thyrotoxic exophthalmos
209. Ans. — C. High myopia

There is usually myopic crescent, chorioretinal atrophy, macular atrophy, vitreous degeneration, retinal detachment, Forster-Fuch's spot and nuclear cataract.

210. Ans. — B. Steroid induced glaucoma
211. Ans. — B. Lenticonus
212. Ans. — D. Hypopituitarism
213. Ans. — D. Toxoplasmosis
214. Ans. — A. Photocoagulates
215. Ans. — B. Presents in the third or fourth decade
216. Ans. — A. Arteriovenous malformations
217. Ans. — E. Mitral regurgitation
218. Ans. — A. Weil-Marchesani syndrome
219. Ans. — C. Ehlers-Danlos syndrome
220. Ans. — D. Autosomal dominant inheritance
221. Ans. — A. HLA B27 states
222. Ans. — B. Corticosteroids
223. Ans. — D. Keratoconus
224. Ans. — B. 6
225. Ans. — A. Homatropine

226. Ans.— A. Hemangioma of choroid and glaucoma

227. Ans.— A. Keratoconjunctivitis

228. Ans.— A. Ciliary groove

229. Ans.— A. Meningioma

230. Ans.— D. Pilocarpine

231. Ans.— A. Strong alkali base

232. Ans.— A. Post. vitreous haemorrhage

233. Ans.— C. Lacrimal gland

234. Ans.— C. 1.49

235. Ans.— C. Retinal detachment

236. Ans.— C. Concussion injury

Berlin's oedema or Commotio retinae occur as a result of blow on the eye. Retinal oedema appears at the posterior pole in the form of milky white cloudiness. Oedema disappears after sometime but central vision remains defective due to chorioretinal degeneration.

237. Ans.— A. Chloroquine

There is high incidence of cotton wool spots, retinal haemorrhages, cytomegalovirus retinitis and conjunctival Kaposi's sarcoma have been described frequently.

238. Ans.— B. Cottonwool spots

239. Ans.— B. Toxoplasmosis

240. Ans.— C. Internal carotid artery ligation

241. Ans.— B. Medial wall

242. Ans.— A. Glaucoma

243. Ans.— B. Dislocation of lens

244. Ans.— B. Macular edema

245. Ans.— B. Excimer laser

246. Ans.— B. Difference in the image size (retinal image).

Upto 5% aniseikonia is well tolerated. The clinical types are optical, retinal and cortical. Symptoms are asthenopia, diplopia and difficulty in depth perception. Optical aniseikonia may be corrected by aniseikonic glasses, contact lenses or intraocular lenses. In retinal aniseikonia, treat the cause and cortical type is very difficult to treat.

247. Ans.— A. Lateral geniculate body

248. Ans.— B. After cataract

249. Ans.— D. Frontal mucocele

250. Ans.— B. 3-5 mm

251. Ans.— C. Autoclaving

252. Ans.— B. Bacterial

253. Ans.— D. Avulsion of optic nerve

254. Ans.— A. Aluminium

255. Ans.— A. Oculomotor palsy

256. Ans.— B. Evisceration

257. Ans.— A. EOG

258. Ans.— C. Lanatoprost

259. Ans.— B. Oculomotor palsy

260. Ans.— B. Cone dystrophy

261. Ans.— C. Most common anomaly is blue green defect.

262. Ans.— A. Protanomaly

In Protanopes, red end of spectrum is much less bright than normal people and is often actually shortened.

263. Ans.— B. Pseudo-papilloedema

264. Ans.— A. Horner's Syndrome

265. Ans.— B. Copper

266. Ans.— B. Panophthalmitis

267. Ans.— A. Retinal detachment

268. Ans.— C. Optic nerve glioma

269. Ans.— A. Enucleation

270. Ans.— B. Retinoblastoma

271. Ans.— B. 3-4 weeks after delivery

272. Ans.— D. Indirect ophthalmoscopy

273. Ans.— D. Squamous blephritis

274. Ans.— C. Buphthalmos

275. Ans.— C. In the capsular bag

276. Ans.— A. The sample should be kept at 4 Degrees C

277. Ans.— A. Enucleation

278. Ans.— C. 6-8 wks

* An artificial eye of plastic should not be worn less than two weeks after exicision. A small eye may be worn for an hour or two a day until the conjunctiva becomes used to the foreign body. Eight or nine weeks after the operation a full sized eye may be worn. A plastic eye need only be taken out & washed once a week.

279. Ans.— B. Age of 15 years

LASIK is only done after the age of 25-30 years when the power of Eye become stable.

280. Ans. — A. Retinoblastoma

281. Ans. — A. Buphthalmos

282. Ans. — A. Rheumatoid arthritis

283. Ans. — A. Optic neuritis

284. Ans. — B. Open angle glaucoma

285. Ans. — A. Yellow

286. Ans. — D. Trachoma

The trachomatous scar may be localised or diffuse. A fine linear scar appears in the sulcus subtarsalis known as Arlt's line.

Trachoma :

- Caused by chlamydia trachomatis.
- Insidious onset, after an incubation period of 5-15 days.
- The symptoms include foreign body sensation, watering, itching photophobia and redness.
- Follicles is the characteristic lesion of trachoma.
- The follicle is invaded by multinucleated macrophage (Laber's cells).
- Typical follicles (Herbet's follicles) may develop on the limbus.
- Follicles leave an oval or circular pits (Herbert's peripheral pits) at limbus, are highly pathognomonic of trachoma
- Pannus may be progressive or regressive.

287. Ans. — D. 1 lack units IM on day 0, 1 and 14

288. Ans. — D. Glaucoma

White pupillary reflex

- Also k/a Amaurotic cats eye reflex or leukocoria

Causes :

- Retinoblastoma
- Congenital cataract
- Retrolental fibroplasia (Retinopathy of prematuritic)
- Persistent hyperplastic primary vitreous
- Inflammatory deposits in eye
- Coloboma of the choroid
- Toxocara endophthalmitis
- Exudative retinopathy of coats
- Tuberculoma of choroid
- Retinal detachment

289. Ans. — B. Wilson disease

290. Ans. — B. Increasing uveoscleral outflow

Latanoprost :

- It is prostaglanding F2 analog
- It lowers the IOP by increasing the aqueous outflow through the uveoscleral pathway.
- Latenoprost (0.005%) is used topically once a day preferably in the evening.
- It is as effective or better than timolol (0.5%) in lowering the IOP.
- Side effect of latanoprost-superficial punctate keratopathy, increased iris pigmentation and cystoid macular oedema.

291. Ans. — B. Leber's hereditary optic neuropathy

Leber's hereditary optic neuropathy

- Laber's hereditary optic neuropathy was the first human disease linked to inherited point mutations in mitochondrial DNA.
- It is a form of retrobulbar neuritis and manifest as painless, subacute, bilateral visual loss with central scotomas and abnormal colour vision.
- A deficiency of cyanocobalamine has been implicated is its etiology.
- Pseudoedema of disc, circumpapillary telangiectasis and nonleakage of fluorescein from telangiectatic vessels constitute the classical triad of it.

292. Ans. — D. Wet AMD (age related macular degeneration)

Photodynamic therapy (PDT) :

- It consists of two essential components, the photosensitizer (dye) that accumulates in the target tissue and a specific laser light corresponding to the absorption peak of the dye.
- Benzoporphysin derivative, verteporfin, and a diode laser are used in PDT to treat the choroidal neovascular membrane of age related macular degeneration (AMD).

293. Ans. — B. Central serous retinopathy

Central serous retinopathy is often transient condition and tends to resolve leaving minute yellow deposits in deeper layers.

294. Ans. — C. Congenital dacryocystitis

Epiphora

- Watering from eye may be due to hypersecretion, failure of lacrimal pump or obstruction of lacrimal passage
- The obstruction of lacrimal passage is the most common cause of epiphora.

Congenital Dacryocystitis

- Due to non-canalisation of the lower end of nasolacrimal duct, usually near the valve of Hasner.
- The condition may be bilateral and manifests as epiphora in newborn.
- Later, purulent discharge develops resulting in matting of eyelashes.
- A gentle pressure over the lacrimal sac produces the reflux of purulent discharge from the lower punctum (regurgitation)

Note: All other condition does not show regurgitation.

295. Ans. — D. Ectopia lentis

Marfan's Syndrome is characterized by a triad.

1. Long, thin extremities with other skeletal changes.
2. Ectopia lentis
3. Aortic aneurysm (esp. at base of aorta)
   - The occular globe is frequently elongated, most patients are myopic and some develop retinal detachment.

296. Ans. — B. Papilloedema

297. Ans. — B. Retinoblastoma

CT findings of Retinoblastoma :

* Gross involvement of optic nerve
* Orbital and CNS involvement
* Pinealoblastoma and CALCIFICATION
* Common age group for Retinoblastoma : *First few years of life or within 2 yr. (seldom seen after 3 years).*
* Both bilateral or unilateral presentation.
* White pupillary reflex : commonest presentation (60%).

1. Coasts disease :
   - usually unilateral
   - First decade (avg. 5 year)
   - visual loss, strabismus
   - white pupillary reflex
   - subretinal exudation (Advanced case), with cholesterol crystals.
   - Flourescin Angiography : Vascular abnormalities and blockage of background fluorescence by hard exudate.

298. Ans. — A. Vitreous haemorrhage

This is a case of vitreous haemorrhage; as suggested by characteristic signs and symptoms as follows :

Symptoms :

* Sudden onset of floaters to significant loss of vision.
* Blurring of vision with a red haze

Signs :

* In mild cases, there may not be any sign of ophthalmoscopically.
* In moderate to severe cases - The fundus cannot be visualized with an ophthalmoscope.
* No fundal glow is visible by distant direct ophthalmoscopy by a plane mirror.

Aetiology

1. Retinal break due to trauma or by vitreous traction.
2. Rupture of newly formed blood vessels
   a. Eale's disease
   b. Retinal venous obstruction
   c. Proliferative diabetic retinopathy
   d. Sickle cell retinopathy
   e. Retinopathy of prematurity
3. Operative - Due to rebleeding following ocular surgery like retiocryopexy.
4. Terson's syndrome :

So, as clearly seen that barring trauma as a cause in this case, there are many other factors which could lead to vitreous haemorrhage.

About other options :

* *Optic atrophy*

- Impairment of colour vision (red-green).
- Relative afferent pupillary defect.
- Ophthalmoscopically
a. Pallor of disc
b. Margins may be sharply defined (in primary optic atrophy) or, blurred (secondary) or less sharply defined (consecutive) Hence, no absence of fundal glow.

* *Developmental cataract :*
  - Known as congenital cataract.
  - It presents at birth or develops soon after birth. So, we could discard this option at this point only, as the patient in question is a 25 yr. old man.
* *Acute attack of angle closure glaucoma :*
  - Acute, intense, unbearable pain radiating along the distribution of 5th cranial nerve.
  - Marked dimness of vision.
  - Redness, lacrimation and photophobia.

In the ques. the patient presents with painless loss of vision.

299. Ans. — D. Cycloplegia

Horner's syndrome consists of :

1. Miosis
2. Partial ptosis
3. Enophthalmos
4. Sometimes, unilateal absence of Sweating of the face on the affected side.
5. Anhydrosis

* In congenital form, there may be heterochromia of the iris.
* IT arises from the damage of sympathetic innervation of the eye.

300. Ans. — A. Trachoma

SAFE strategy for trachoma in vision 2020 programme :

S = Surgery for trichiasis/entropion

A=Antibiotics

F= Facial cleanliness

E = Environmental sanitation

301. Ans. — B. Circulus iridis major

Hyphaema due to injury

Without any tear → Source of bleeding → Small branches of the circulus iridis major due to tear between longitudinal and circular fibres of the ciliary muscle

With tear of sphincter → Source of bleeding → Capillaries of the circulus iridis minor

* If there is iridodialysis: Radial vessels at the iris root source of bleeding).

302. Ans. — D. Dopamine

303. Ans. — B. IL-8

* In vivo angiogenesis in corneal or chorioallantoic membrane models induced by *basic fibroblast growth factor* or by *tumor necrosis factor-depended* on, whereas angiogenesis initiated by *vascular endothelial growth factor*, transforming growth factor, or phorbol ester depended on.

304. Ans. — A. Spares ocular muscle

* LEMS is a presynaptic disorder of the neuro-muscular junction that can cause weakness similar to that of MG.
* The proximal muscles of the lower limbs are most commonly affected, but other muscles may be involved as well.

305. Ans. — B. Pars plana vitrectomy

Vitrectomy is the treatment of choice for vitro macular traction which if left would lead to retinal detachement. It involves removing the cloudy vitreous and replacing it with a silicon oil.

Bevacizumab is anti-VEGF antibody. Blocking Vascular endothelial growth factor (VEGF) prevents angiogenesis, but has no role in treating macular traction.

Laser photocoagulation uses the heat from the laser to seal or destroy abnormal, leaking blood vessels in the retina. It is not effective to treat macular traction.

306. Ans. — B. Laser photocoagulatin of both eyes

The hallmark of retinopathy of prematurity (ROP) is abnormal retinal vasculature. Ophthalmologists diagnose and make decision about the initial treatment of ROP based on the appearence of the retinal blood vessels. "Plus" disease. It is a sign of rapidly progressive ROP and is indication for early laser ablation of the peripheral avascular retina.

Threshold disease : It is defined as stage 3+ ROP in zones 1 or 2 occupying at least five contiguous clock hours or eight noncontiguous clock hours of retina.

Treatment of threshold disease is laser photocoagulation.

Prethreshold disease is divided into 2 types :

High risk or type-I treatment is laser photocoagulation

Low risk or type II- treatment is weekly or twice weekly observation

Type I prethreshold	Type-II prethreshold
Zone I ROP (any stage) Zone I, stage 3 Zone II, stage 2/3 +	Zone I, stage 1/2 Zone II, stage 3
Laser photocoagulation	Weekly or twice weekly observation

In this question the child with zone 1, stage II plus ROP falls into prethreshold disease. Type I or high risk type, hence laser photocoagulation would be the management of choice.

307. Ans. — D. Functional visual loss

Since papillary reaction is afected in optic neuritis, fundus cannot be normal in AION and CMV Retinitis, hence diagnosis of exclusion is functional vision loss which is known to show normal ocular features on examination.

308. Ans. — B. Post ganglionic sympathetic fibres from Edinger Westphal nucleus

Dilator pupilac is supplied with nonmyelinated post ganglionic fibers from the superior sympathetic ganglion.

Dilator Pupillae is supplied by adrenergic fibers of cervical sympathetic nerves. The dilator tract probably commences in hypothalamus not far from constrictor centre and also has connection with cerebral cortex.

309. Ans. — C. Oguchi's disease

The fundus oculi presents a most peculiar appearance. The posterior pole and in many cases the whole of fundus, instead of having a normal orange-red colour, presents a curious shining greyish-pink background, on which the retinal vessels stand out sharply. The vessels appear dark with little distinction between the arteries and the veins. The finer divisions of the blood vessels can be easily followed to their finest ramifications. At places a dark shadow or a bright white line may be seen alongside the blood vessel.

The most interesting feature of this disease in well marked cases is the reversal of all the feature sdescribed above, if the patient sits in the dark for about one hour. This is called Mizuo's phenomenon.

Stargardt disease, or fundus flavimaculatus, is an inherited juvenile macular degeneration that causes progressive vision loss usually to the point of legal blindness. The progression usually starts between the ages of six and twelve years old and plateaus shortly after rapid reduction in visual acuity.

Fundus Albipunctatus

A disorder in which gray or white mottling of the fundus of the eye is associated with night blindness; cassed also Lauber disease.

310. Ans. — C. Pharmacological blockade

* In Adie pupil there is denervation hypersensitivity and hence the pupil reacts even with very low dose of pilocarpine.
* In diabetic 3rd nerve palsy there will be pupillary sparing whereas
* In uncal herniation there will be surgical 3rd nerve palsy, hence pupillary fibres will be involved but it should react to pilocarpine.

Pharmacological blockade indicates that patient has used a mydriatic and hence there is no action of pilocarpine

311. Ans. — A. Nerve cells

It selectively affects retal cells or putamen cells. Ethanol blocks competitively. 6/18 in best eye — Normal

6/18 to 6/60 in best eye—Low vision

Cannot see 6/60 but can see 3/60—Economical blindness

Cannot see 3/60 but can see 1/60—Social blindness

Cannot see 1/60 but can see light—manifest blindness

Undetermined—Absolute blindness

312. Ans. — A. Symblepharon

Alkali substances are lipophilic and penetrate more rapidly. In mild caes there erosion, is moderate corneal opacity and in severe avascularly of limbus. Conjunctival scarring, symblepharon or ankyloblepharon, cataract or phthisis bulbi can result.

313. Ans. — D. Preliferative retinopathy

Peripheral retina is affected. It is also called periphlebitis retinae and angiopathia retinae juvenalis 20-30 year of age.

314. Ans. — A. Topicamide

Mydriatics

		Concentration	*Duration*
A.	Atropine	0.5-2	2 weeks
B.	Oxyphenonium	1-5	12 days
C.	Hyoscine	0.25-0.5	5 days
D.	Eucatropine	5-10	4 hours
E.	Cyclopentolate	0.5-2	24 hours
F.	Topicamide	1-2	6 hours
G.	Lachesine	1-2	6 hours

315. Ans. — B. Osteosarcoma

Repeat Question.

316. Ans. — A. Pathological myopia

Repeat Question.

317. Ans. — A. Nd-Yag laser

Important Question. LASIK (Laser assisted in situ keratomileusis) and PRK (Photorefractive heratectomy) or ASA (Advanced surface ablation) are used.

318. Ans. — A. Papilloedema

Repeat Question.. Retinal detachment and CRAO are other causes.

319. Ans. — A. Open angle glaucoma

Repeat Question.

320. Ans. — A. Reiter's disease

Repeat Question. Knee and sacroiliac joints are most commonly affected.

321. Ans. — B. Cervix

Repeat Question.

322. Ans. — B. High myopia

Repeat Question.

323. Ans. — C. Sympathetic ophthalmia

324. Ans. — C. Cotton wool spots

Repeat Question.

325. Ans. — B. VII

Schirmer's test

Normal : more than 14 mm ; wetting of paper after 5 min.

Mild : 14-9 mm ; wetting of paper after 5 min.

Moderate : 8-4 mm ; wetting of paper after 5 min.

Severe : less than 4 mm ; wetting of paper after 5 min.

326. Ans. — C. Vitamin A deficiency

Childhood blindness, trachoma, corneal blindness and glaucoma also included.

327. Ans. — B. Pigmendary retinal dystrophy

It is seen in retinitis pigmentosa. It can be AD (Autosomal dominant), AR or X-linked.

328. Ans. — A. DM

Read text for causes. Important one are HT, DM, cardiac valvular lesions, patent foramen ovale, embolism, atherosclerosis, giant cell arteritis, hypercoagulable states, collagen vascular ds , OCP, polycythemia, PAN and rarely Behcet's syndrome, syphilis, sickle cell ds and migraine.

REVIEW PAPER-I

(Based on Difficult & Important MCQ's)

1. **Asthenopia is typically seen in :**
   A. Miners B. Pilots
   C. Watch makers D. Sea explorers
2. **Atkinson block is —— nerve block :**
   A. II B. III
   C. VI D. VII
3. **Beilschowsky's test is used to identify :**
   A. Angle closure glaucoma
   B. Congenital cataract
   C. Paretic cyclovertical muscle
   D. Severe myopia
4. **Blessing-Iwanoff cysts are seen in :**
   A. Macular degeneration
   B. Hypermature cataract
   C. Follicular conjunctivitis
   D. Normal Elderly
5. **Egger's line is seen between :**
   A. Cornea and aqueous
   B. Aqueous and ant. lens capsule
   C. Post lens capsule and ant. hyaloid
   D. Vitreous and retina
6. **Hyalocytes are seen in :**
   A. Aqueous B. Vitreous
   C. Sclera D. Retina
7. **Hughes's procedure is used to :**
   A. Reconstruct upper lid defects
   B. Reconstruct lower lid defects
   C. Correct congenital glaucoma
   D. Treat diabetic retinopathy
8. **Jones test is used to detect :**
   A. Angle closure glaucoma
   B. Lens dislocation
   C. Patency of nasolacrimal du
   D. Vitreous opacities
9. **Iridoplegia in most commonly seen following :**
   A. Diabetes mellitus B. III nerve palsy
   C. Trauma D. Congenital defect
10. **Irvine-Gas defect follows :**
    A. Mydriatic use B. Cataraqct surgery
    C. Hypertension D. Pupillary oedema
11. **Jensen procedure is preformed to correct deformity following ——— nerve palsy :**
    A. III B. IV
    C. VI D. VII
12. **Krimsky test is used for :**
    A. Astigmatism B. Buphthalmos
    C. Strabismus D. Immature cataract
13. **Knapp's rule is used for :**
    A. Anosocoria B. Anisometropia
    C. Asthenopia D. Lenticonus
14. **Purkinje shift is typically seen from a maximum of ——— nm under photopic conditions to—— nm maximum under scotopic conditions :**
    A. 555 to 510 B. 585 to 555
    C. 510 to 430 D. 430 to 390
15. **Uhthoff's sign is seen in :**
    A. Diabetic retinopathy
    B. Demyelinating optic neuritis
    C. Craniopharyngioma
    D. Diabetes insipidus
16. **Absorption and Emision peaks on Fluorescein angiography are respectively :**
    A. 465-490,520-530 B. 435-465,465-485
    C. 410-425,435-465 D. 395-415,430-445
17. **Fleurette is seen in :**
    A. Melanoma B. Retinoblastoma
    C. Galactosemia D. Diabetes mellitus
18. **Term "A" pattern is used in :**
    A. Retinopathy
    B. Field defects in glaucoma
    C. Strabismus
    D. Radiation injury
19. **Barkan's membrane is seen on :**
    A. Conjunctiva B. Cornea
    C. Trabecular sheet D. Retina

Ans.									
1. C	2. D	3. C	4. B	5. C	6. B	7. B	8. C	9. C	10. B
11. C	12. C	13. B	14. A	15. B	16. A	17. B	18. C	19. C	

20. **Bear tracks are seen on :**
A. Cornea B. Sclera
C. Vitreous D. Retina

21. **Worth's four dot test is used for following except :**
A. For near and distance
B. Monofixation syndrome (Microtropia)
C. Anomalous retinal correspondence (ARC)
D. Diplopia

22. **Worth four dot test subtends (on the macula) an angle of —— for near and —— for distance :**
A. 4.5,6.0 B. 6.0, 1.5
C. 4.0, 2.0 D. 8.0, 1.5

23. **The following test is used to test stereopsis except :**
A. Worth's four dot test B. Synoptophore
C. Bar reading D. Bagolini striated glasses

24. **True about Faden (post fixation sutures) are all except :**
A. Non-absorbabale and permanent
B. Temproary
C. Used on recti muscles
D. Indicated in dissociated vertical deviation

25. **Protein content of lens is higher than any organ in the body and is — %**
A. 10 B. 16
C. 33 D. 60

26. **The abundant neurotroansmitter in retina is:**
A. Substance -P B. Noradrenaline
C. Acetylcholine D. Serotonin

27. **Vitamin A deficiency may be caused by renal disease due to :**
A. metabolism by liver B. Protein binding
C. Storage D. Excretion

28. **In human retina, rod density is maximum —— mm from fovea**
A. 1 B. 2.5
C. 4 D. 6

29. **In human retina, there are —— million rods and — million cones:**
A. 60, 30 B. 100 ,3
C. 120 ,6 D. 90 ,20

30. **In optic nerve, the upper limit of normal VER latency is ——— m sec :**
A. 8 B. 100
C. 115 D. 135

31. **Normal cup size in optic disc is :**
A. 0.1-0.2 B. 0.2-0.3
C. 0.3-0.4 D. 0.5-0.6

32. **Hassal-Henle's bodies are seen in ——— degeneration of cornea :**
A. Amyloid B. Senile
C. Calcific D. Hyaline

33. **Choroidal metastatic tumor most commonly arises from :**
A. Lymph nodes B. Bronchus
C. Nai D. GI tract

34. **Following test is normal in retinits pigmentosa :**
A. Photopic ERG B. Scotopic ERG
C. VER D. EOG

35. **The following structures are mesodermal in origin except :**
A. Iris storma B. Levator palpebrae
C. Dilator muscle of iris D. Ciliary muscle

36. **Cornea has an average central thicknes of—— mm :**
A. 0.46 B. 0.56
C. 0.66 D. 0.76

37. **Stroma constitutes——— % of normal corneal thickness :**
A. 50 B. 60
C. 75 D. 90

38. **The ratio of crossed to uncrossed fibres in the optic chiasma is :**
A. 75 :25 B. 63 : 37
C. 53 : 47 D. 50 : 50

39. **Uveal melanocytes develop from :**
A. Surface ectoderm B. Neuroectoderm
C. Neural crest cells D. Endothelium

40. **Hyaloid vascular system disappears in the ——— months of foetal life :**
A. 5 B. 6
C. 7 D. 8

41. **Blood flow in hyaloid vascular system disappears by ——— month :**
A. 5 B. 6
C. 7 D. 8

42. **Latent period in photoophthalmia is——— hours :**
A. 1-2 B. 4-5
C. 10-12 D. 24-30

43. **Thygeson's superficial punctate keratitis is characterized by following except :**
A. Snow flake epithelial lesions
B. Conjunctivitis associated
C. Granular gray dots in early lesion
D. Responsive to steroids

Ans.									
20. D	21. D	22. B	23. B	24. B	25. C	26. C	27. D	28. D	29. C
30. C	31. C	32. B	33. B	34. A	35. C	36. B	37. D	38. C	39. C
40. D	41. C	42. B	43. B						

44. A sterile immune ring (yellow line of demorcation) is typically seen in :
A. Trachoma
B. Herpetic corneal ular
C. Mycotic corneal ular
D. Phlyctenular keratitis

45. Lucid interval of Vogt is seen in :
A. Diabetic retinopathy
B. Photo ophthalmia
C. Sympathetic ophthalmia
D. Arcus senilis

46. Commonest senile change seen in cornea is :
A. Arcus juvenilis
B. Arcus senilis
C. Vogt's white limbal girdle
D. Hassal-Henle bodies

47. True about congenital glaucoma are except :
A. Over 65% boys
B. Over 75% unilateral
C. Incidence 1 in 1000
D. Autosomal recessive inheritance

48. Large cup is defined as size of ——— or more :
A. 0.4 B. 0.5
C. 0.6 D. 0.3

49. Cornea guttata is seen in :
A. Lipid keratopathy
B. Hassal-Henle bodies
C. Band keratopathy
D. Salzmann's nodular degeneration

50. In optic disc changes in primary open glaucoma, a difference of more than ——— between 2 eyes is significant :
A. 0.61 B. 0.02
C. 0.1 D. 0.2

51. Features of Keratoacanthoma include all except :
A. Seen more commonly in elderly
B. Has dense infiltrate of bassophils
C. Crater shaped
D. May regress

52. Extreme photophobia is characteristic of all of the following except :
A. Mycotic keratitis B. Aniridia
C. Cystinosis D. Acanthameoba Keratitis

53. Following are true about Terrien's disease except :
A. Is bilateral
B. Visual impairment due to astigmatism
C. Is painless
D. Elderly females affected

54. Giant conjunctival papillae occur in :
A. Adenovirus conjunctivites
B. Mycotic
C. Acanthamoeba infection
D. Ocular prosthesis wear

55. Filamentary keratitis is seen in all except :
A. Herpes Zoster Katitis
B. Keratoconjunctives sicca
C. Amiodarone keratoconjunctivitis
D. Supreior limbal keratoconjunctivitis

56. Recurrent corneal erosions occur in all except :
A. Reis Bucklers dystrophy
B. Lattica dystrophy
C. Granular dystrophy
D. Microcystic dystrophy

57. Climatic keratopathy is due to cummulative exposure to :
A. U-V ligh B. Infrard light
C. Heat D. Cold

58. Surgical procedures used in the mangement of malignant melonoma of conjunctivia include all except :
A. Enucleation
B. Exanteration
C. Cryo therapy
D. Diathermy

59. Cornea obtains glucose mainly from :
A. Aqueous B. Tear film
C. Limbal capillaries D. Sclera

60. Corneal endothelium obtains most of its oxygen from :
A. Aqueous B. Tear film
C. Limbal capillaries D. Air

61. The variations of intraocular pressure with arterial pulse is ± —— mmHg :
A. 1.0 B. 2.0
C. 2.5 D. 3.0

62. The variations of intraocular pressure with phases of respiration ———mmHg:
A. 1 B. 2
C. 3 D. 3.5

63. At the onset of sleep, intraocular pressure — :
A. Decreases slowly B. Increases slowly
C. Decreases rapidly D. Increases rapidly

64. The total volume of vitreous pressure in both the globes is ——— ml :
A. 5.2 B. 6.4
C. 7.8 D. 9.6

Ans. 44. C 45. D 46. D 47. B 48. C 49. B 50. D 51. B 52. A 53. D
54. D 55. C 56. C 57. A 58. D 59. A 60. A 61. A 62. A 63. C
64. C

65. Lens contains —times— content of K+ than aqueous humor :

A. 15, lower B. 15, higher
C. 25, lowe D. 25, higher

66. Blpharophimosis syndrome is :

A. Autosomal dominant B. Autosomal recassive
C. X- linked dominant D. X- linked recessive

67. The Marcus Gunn jaw-winking phenomenon is a cause of ———which varies with movement of jaw :

A. Diplopia B. Nystagmus
C. Ptosis D. Enophthalmos

68. Marcus Gunn jaw-winking phenomenon is a due to synkinesis between levator palpabrae superiors and ——:

A. Masster B. Zygomaticus
C. Pterygoid D. Digastric

69. The Fasanella-Servat operation is used in correction of ptosis in which levator function exceeds——— mm :

A. 1- B. 3-5
C. 5-10 D. 15-20

70. Before levator muscle resection in ptosis, prior to surgery, at least——— mm levator function should be present :

A. 1 B. 4
C. 10 D. 15

71. A levator muscle resection, for 5 mm of levator function, resect——— mm of muscle :

A. 5- B. 8-12
C. 14-18 D. 22-26

72. In Leber's congenital amaurosis, the diagnosis is made on the basis of abnormal :

A. VER B. EOG
C. ERG D. All of the above

73. In Best's macular dystrophy, following are true except :

A. Autosomal dominant
B. EOG is electrodiagnostic test of choice
C. ERG abnormalities in carriers
D. EOG is abnormal long before visual acquity falls

74. The following are correct finding on Snellen visual acquity chart except :

A. <6/60 in arteritic ischaemic optic neuropathy
B. 6/6 in melanocytoma of optic disc
C. 6/60 in central serous choriodopathy
D. 6/6 in tyrosinase positive occulocutaneous albinism

75. Pavingstone degeneration is most commonly seen in :

A. Uveal melanom B. Retinitis pigmentosa
C. Harada's disease D. Normal eyes

76. Following are correct about persistent hyperplastic primary vitreous (PHPV) except :

A. PHPV typically occurs in microphthalmos
B. PHPV is usually unilateral in 90%
C. Ciliary processes are abnormal
D. Prognosis for vision is good in anterior PHPV

77. Argon laser photocoagulation is beneficial in following diabetic maculopathy except :

A. Ischaemic B. Exudative
C. Oedematou D. None of the above

78. Following are true about Drusen except :

A. Secondary calcification
B. ERG changes
C. Peripapillary haemorrhage
D. RPE changes

79. Following drugs may cause benign intracranial hypertension except :

A. Corticosteroids B. Ethambutol
C. Vitamin A D. Nalidixic acid

80. 'Ganda' is a combination of :

A. Sulfamethoxazole & Gentamicin
B. Penicillin & Streptomycin
C. Guenethidine & Adrenaline
D. Phenylephrine & Pilocarpine

81. Batten-Mayou disease has onset at the age of— years :

A. 0-3 B. 3-5
C. 5-8 D. 9-12

82. Badewing is appearance on :

A. Retinoscopy
B. Direct ophthalmoscopy
C. Indirect ophthalmoscopy
D. Slit-lamp examination

83. Behr's sign is :

A. Anisocoria B. Aniridia
C. Anisometropia D. Antimetropia

84. Berger's space is slitlike space between :

A. Aqueous and ant.lens capsule
B. Cornea and aqueous humour
C. Post.lens capsule and vitreous
D. Vitreous and retina

85. The pain in Tolosa Hunt syndrome is best treated with :

A. Atropine B. Corticosteroids
C. Aspirin D. Ciprofloxacin

86. Berman locater is useful in :

A. Congenital glaucoma
B. Congenital cataract
C. Metallic intraocular foreign body
D. Diabetic retinopathy

Ans.										
	65. D	66. A	67. C	68. C	69. C	70. B	71. D	72. C	73. C	74. D
	75. D	76. D	77. A	78. B	79. B	80. C	81. C	82. D	83. A	84. C
	85. B	86. C								

87. **Knoepp's nodules are found in :**
A. Cornea B. Iris
C. Sclera D. Conjunctiva

88. **Lockwood's ligament is a fascial band formed by blending of sheaths of :**
A. Superior oblique and sup. rectus
B. Superior oblique and lateral rectus
C. Inferior oblique and inferior rectus
D. Inferior rectus and lateral rectus

89. **Glands of Manz are seen in :**
A. Retina B. Bulbar conjunctiva
C. Lacrimal apparatus D. Nasolacrimal duct

90. **Busacca nodules are present in :**
A. Trachoma
B. Follicular conjunctivitis
C. Grannulomatous uveitis
D. Non-granulomatous uveitis

91. **Landolt rings are used to test :**
A. Visual acquity B. Color vision
C. IOP D. Vitreous opacities

92. **Knoepp's lens is used in :**
A. Myopia B. Astigmatism
C. Retinopathy D. Gonioscopy

93. **Lyon's hypothesis is used to explain expression of —— disease :**
A. Autosomal dominant B. Autosomal recessive
C. X-linked dominant D. X-linked recessive

94. **Kuhnt-Symanowski procedure is used for :**
A. Ectropion B. Entropion
C. Keratoconus D. Megalocornea

95. **Visual acquity in an infant of 6 months age is :**
A. 20/400 B. 20/200
C. 20/100 D. 20/50

96. **In fetus Angio genesis in eye involve all except :**
A. TNF β B. IL-B
C. BFGF D. VEGF

97. **In maddox rod, the line image seen by the patient is :**
A. Green B. Red
C. Blue D. White

98. **The cross cylinder is used to check the ——-of a cylinderical lens :**
A. Axis B. Power
C. Both D. None of the above

99. **The Stiles-Crawford effect —— ocular —— aberration :**
A. Increases, Chromatic B. Decreases, Chromatic
C. Increases, Spherical D. Decreases, Spherical

100. **To focus an object at 25 cm, the emmetropic must exert —— diopters of accomodative power :**
A. 1 B. 2
C. 4 D. 10

101. **Conjunctival scarring is a feature of the following use except :**
A. Phenobarbitone B. Tetracycline
C. Practolol D. Sulfamethoxazole

102. **After levator muscle resection surgery, a Frost suture is placed in the — lid margin at the end of surgery to protect the cornea for 48 hours :**
A. Upper B. Lower
C. Both D. None of the above

103. **The most common cause of axial proptosis is :**
A. Myopia B. Retinoblastoma
C. Dysthyroid eye disease D. Diabetes mellitus

104. **Features of idiopathic orbital pseudotumor include all except :**
A. Rapid onset & seen in elderly
B. Spontaneous remission
C. Recurrence in contralateral orbit
D. Dramatic response to systemic corticosteroids

105. **Surgery is indicated in blow out fracture if there is :**
A. Any diplopia of > 2 weeks
B. Diplopia in primary position and/or downgaze
C. Diplopia in primary position and/or uppergaze
D. Diplopia in secondary position

106. **Indication of surgery in blowout fracture is indicated if there is enophthalmos greater than —— mm :**
A. 0.5 B. 1.0
C. 1.5 D. 2.0

107. **Saccadic eye movements are controlled by all except :**
A. Cerebellum B. Superior colliculus
C. Temporal cortex D. Posterior commissure

108. **The latency of saccades is —— m sec :**
A. 50-150 B. 100-200
C. 200-250 D. 250-350

109. **The latency of pursuit eye movement is —— msec :**
A. 60 B. 130
C. 180 D. 210

110. **If the diopteric power of the eye in a 4-year old child is 15 D, the power in a20-year old will be — D :**
A. 6 B. 11
C. 18 D. 21

111. **Normal AC/A ratio (A-Accomodation C-Convergence) is —— prism diopters :**
A. 1 B. 2
C. 4 D. 8

Ans. 87. B 88. C 89. B 90. C 91. A 92. D 93. D 94. A 95. B 96. B 97. B 98. C 99. D 100. C 101. B 102. B 103. C 104. A 105. B 106. D 107. C 108. C 109. B 110. B 111. C

112. **Volume of tear film is — ml :**
A. 1-2 B. 3-5
C. 5-10 D. 20-25

113. **Albumin constitutes —— % of protein :**
A. 40 B. 50
C. 60 D. 90

114. **A change of the sign of optical rotation of specimen as the wavelength of observation is changed, the change occurring at the wavelength of an absorption band is called :**
A. Orbelli effect B. Cotton effect
C. Downman effect D. Edison effect

115. **The displacement towards the shorter Wavelength of sensitivity to brightness under condition scotopic, as compared to photopic vision. It explain why blue colour appears relatively brighter in weak light. This is called**
A. Wever Bray effect B. Zeeman effect
C. Stiles- Crawford effect D. Purkinje effect

116. **The phenomenon in which light entering through the center of the pupil appears brighter than the same light when entering through a peripheral part is called :**
A. Tyndall B. Stiles Crawford effect
C. Vulpian effect D. Édison effect

117. **Full dark adaptation takes longer than ——— minutes**
A. 3 B. 5
C. 10 D. 30

118. **Equator is ——— mm from the limbus**
A. 8 B. 10
C. 12 D. 16

119. **In Gopalan syndrome, following visual defects are present except :**
A. Amblyopia B. Central scotoma
C. Paracentral scotoma D. Optic neuritis

120. **Tear breakup time is normal if it is —— sec**
A. 3 B. 5
C. 10 D. 16

121. **Xanthelasma is seen in the following syndromes except :**
A. Bogaert van Scherer Epstein syndrome
B. Hand Schullar Christian syndrome
C. Letter-Siwe syndrome
D. Wagner syndrome

122. **Spherophakia is seen in the following except :**
A. Achard syndrome B. Marchesani syndrome
C. Homocystinuria D. Herrick syndrome
E. Marfan syndrome

123. **Pseudoglioma is seen in the following syndrome :**
A. Bloch- Sulzberger B. Caffey
C. Folling D. Naegeli

124. **Normal tear meniscus is approximately —— mm in height**
A. 0.2 B. 0.5
C. 1.0 D. 1.5

125. **Normal value on Schirmer I test is ——mm :**
A. 1-10 B. 10-20
C. 20-30 D. Above 30

126. **Hperfluoresscene from optic disc with neovascularization is seen in :**
A. Cystoid macular oedema
B. Hemangioma
C. Papillitis
D. Diabetes mellitus

127. **In Prone Provocative test for angle closure glaucoma, a rise of intraocular pressure of at least —— mm Hg is considered positive :**
A. 2-4 B. 4-6
C. 8-10 D. 15-18

128. **Flexner- Wintersteiner rossettes are seen in :**
A. Diabetic retinopathy
B. Chloroquine induced retinopathy
C. Retinoblastoma
D. Pseudoglioma

129. **Flieringa ring is used in some intraocular procedures to avoid :**
A. Rise in IOP B. Scleral collapse
C. Corneal opacity D. Lens dislocation

130. **Maximum visual acquity is seen in :**
A. Fleurette B. Fovea
C. Foveola D. Ferry's line

131. **The range of saccadic eye movement, is ——— degrees/ sec :**
A. 30-700 B. 60-600
C. 90-900 D. 120-1200

132. **Hypermetropic or myopic spherical errors of > 4 are —— corrected to 6/6 with a pin hole :**
A. Alway B. Sometimes
C. Rarely D. Not

133. **In retinoscopy at 0.66 m, the correction for working distances is ——— D :**
A. 0.46 B. 0.66
C. 1.5 D. 3.5

134. **The diopteric power of Hruby lens is ——— D :**
A. 15.6 B. 26.4
C. 48.2 D. 58.6

135. **The area of contact of Goldmann's applanation tonometer is ——— mm in diameter :**
A. 2.16 B. 3.06
C. 4.26 D. 4.76

Ans. 112. C 113. C 114. B 115. D 116. B 117. D 118. D 119. D 120. C 121. D
122. D 123. A 124. C 125. B 126. D 127. C 128. C 129. B 130. C 131. A
132. D 133. C 134. D 135. B

136. Which of the following is false :
A. A patient with 3D myopia has a far point at 33 cm
B. In a patient with axial myopia of 19 D, emmetropia will result from lens extraction
C. A patient with 3 D hypermetropia needs to exert 1 D of accomodation to see image in 2 eyes
D. Aniseikonia is a difference in retinal image in 2 eyes

137. Aqueous contains higher contents of the following than plasma :
A. Albumin B. Globulins
C. Vitamin B1 D. Vitamin C

138. ———— Stain is used in the diagnosis of mascular dystrophy :
A. Masson's trichome B. PAS
C. Methylene blue D. ZN

139. Features of primary open angle glaucoma include the following except :
A. Posterior displacement of lamina cribrosa
B. Widening of pial septa in the optic nerve
C. Photorreceptor loss
D. Ganglion cell loss

140. In sarcoidosis, conjunctival nodules are :
A. Purple B. Blue
C. Orange D. Red

141. "Essential shrinkage" of conjunctiva is typically seen in :
A. Leprosy
B. Tularemia
C. Oculocutaneous syndrome
D. Irritative conjunctivitis

142. In aphakia anterior focal point becomes ——— mm in front of cornea :
A. 21.4 B. 23.2
C. 27.3 D. 31

143. True about tuberculoma of conjunctiva are following except :
A. Palpebral conjunctiva is involved
B. Bulbar conjunctiva is involved
C. Ulcerative lesion
D. Hard nodular

144. True about opthalmia nodosa is except :
A. Is due to irritation caused by retained hair of cater pillar
B. May be mistaken for tubercular nodules
C. Histology reveals hair surrounded by neutriphils and eosinophils
D. Excision biopsy is the treatment

145. Following fungi are commonly responsible for mycotic corneal ulcers except :
A. Candida B. Aspergillus
C. Fusarium D. Histoplasma

146. Chlamydia trachomatis serotypes D-K cause all of the following except :
A. Ophthalamia neonatorum B. Trachoma
C. Non-specific urethritis D. Adult inclusion

147. 30 minutes following instillation conjunctivitis into the normal eye of an emmetropic 20-year-old there is mydraisis and the near point of accomodation is 10 cm. The drop could be :
A. Gunethidine B. Physostigmine
C. Cyclopentolate D. Phenylephrine

148. Inhibition of which enzyme reduces cataract formation in diabetes mellitus :
A. Galactose kinase B. Tyrosinase
C. Aldose reductase D. Cyclooxygenase

149. Following are true about recession except
A. Medial rectus has greater effect than recession of lateral rectus
B. A vertical muscle has a greater effect than recession of horizontal muscle
C. Bilateral lateral recti recession is indicated in divergence insufficiency esodeviation
D. Conjunctiva decrease the effect of muscle recession

150. True about adjustable suture surgery is all except :
A. The maximum recession necessary is initially performed so that adjustment will involve readvancement
B. More sutiable for vertical than horizontal recti
C. Suitable in children
D. Suitable for consecutive exotropia

Ans. **136. C** **137. D** **138. B** **139. C** **140. C** **141. C** **142. B** **143. C** **144. C** **145. D**
146. B **147. D** **148. C** **149. D** **150. C**

QUICK MEDICAL TEXT REVIEW SERIES

About this Series

- Comprehensive collection of **Important Text** subjectwise arranged
- This series include 20 books of Anatomy, Biochemistry, Physiology, Pharmacology, Microbiology, Forensic Medicine, Pathology, SPM, General Medicine, Psychiatry, Dermatology, Pediatrics, General Medicine, Orthopaedics, Anaesthesia, Ophthalmology, ENT, Gynaecology, Obstetrics and Radiology.
- Each book has been contributed by an *expert examiner of his field*
- This series is cost-effective supplement to the author's comprehensive book on MCQ's i.e. ***Quick Medical Examinations Review Series*** *(containing 40,000 MCQ's subjectwise)*
- **Important Topics** (for MCQ's and undergraduate examinations) in each subject has been listed in the beginning of each book to stress selective reading.
- There is no need to underline the books for MCQ's because important points to be remembered have been added at the beginning of each chapter.
- The books contains text from many standard textbooks of each subject
- Each book contains many important points and text usually **not covered by standard textbooks**
- Each series is presented with the hope and wish to invite fruitful interaction, comments, suggestions and contributions from its readers.
- Edited by : **Dr. M.S. Bhatia (MD; Dip. W.P.A., MNAMS)** - an experienced teacher and examiner who has worked in three leading Medical Colleges of Delhi (Maulana Azad Medical College, Lady Hardinge Medical College & University College of Medical Sciences) under Delhi University.
- Please send you suggestions and contributions to : **Dr. M.S. Bhatia,** D-1, Naraina Vihar, New Delhi - 110 028.

Keep your knowledge uptodate with this new series from:

CBS Publishers & Distributors Pvt. Ltd.

NEW DELHI • BANGALORE • PUNE • CHENNAI • COCHIN (INDIA)

REVIEW PAPER-II

(Based on Difficult & Important MCQ's)

1. A patient has an amplitude of accomodation of 4.00 diopters. At what distance will he be able to read comfortably ?
A. 25 B. 50 cm
C. 60 cm D. 80 cm

2. Which of the following are "against the rule" keratometry readings :
A. 44.0/44.0 at 90° B. 45.0/45.0 at 180°
C. 44.0/46.0 at 180° D. 43.0/48.0 at 180°

3. Base curves of a lens can be checked with a :
A. Geneva lens measure B. Len caliper
C. Lensometer D. Neutralizing lens

4. Which soluble crystalline protein is maximum in lens :
A. Alpha B. Beta
C. Gamma D. All are equal

5. Attention reflex of pupil is ——— reflex :
A. Oppenheim's B. Philippson's
C. Preyer's D. Piltz's

6. A 4-PD base cut prism is placed in front of a patient's right eye while the patient fixates a target at 6 meters. A small shift of both eyes to the left is seen. This indicates :
A. Convergence insufficiency
B. A non-specific finding
C. Scotoma at macula OD
D. Scrotoma at macula OS

7. The points in the retina which are not paired exactly are ——— points :
A. Corresponding B. Disparate
C. Divergence D. Dispersion

8. Eye Bandage covering both the diseases and the healthy eye is ——— bandage :
A. Buller's B. Barton's
C. Borsch's D. Esmarch's

9. Spatium episclerale is known as ——— space :
A. Tarin's B. Tenon's
C. Zang's D. Kiernan's

10. Small white spots on the periphery of the iris, usually cresenteric, with concavity outward are —— spots :
A. Bitot B. Brushfield
C. Carleton D. Christopher's

11. Bilateral pupillary contraction when the patient sits in the darkened room and without accomodation within the field of vision is —— reflex :
A. Gifford's B. Haab's
C. Joffroy's D. Loven's

12. Keratitis nummularis is also called ——— Keratitis:
A. Lattice B. Dimmer
C. Rosacea D. Trantas

13. Which of the following dots represent the remains of the lenticular attachment of the hyaloid artery :
A. Marcus Gunn's B. Gunn's
C. Mittendorf's D. Trantas

14. Gunn's dots are —— coloured seen about the macula lutea :
A. White] B. Red
C. Blue D. Yellow

15. The operation of which instrument is based on one of the Purkinje-Sanson images :
A. Cross cylinder B. Slit lamp
C. Retinoscope D. Keratometer

16. Glassblower's (heat) Cataract usually beings at the :
A. Ant.Capsular layer B. Nuclear layer
C. "Y" sutures D. Posterior cortical area

17. Orbicularis pupillary reflex is also known as——— reflex :
A. Gault's B. Erben's
C. Escherich's D. Gifford's

18. Oculocardiac reflex is also known as ——— reflex :
A. Abram's B. Aschner's
C. Babkin's D. Barkman's

19. In Brown's syndrome there is failure of :
A. Elevation in adducted eye
B. Elevation in abducted eye
C. Depression in adducted eye
D. Depression in abducted eye

Ans.	1. B	2. C	3. A	4. B	5. D	6. D	7. B	8. C	9. B	10. B
	11. B	12. B	13. C	14. A	15. D	16. D	17. D	18. B	19. A	

20. **In inverse Duane's syndrome, there is limitation of :**
A. Elevation B. Depression
C. Abduction D. Adduction

21. **The syndrome of Wildervanck consists of following except :**
A. Congenital labyrinthine deafness
B. Klippel-Feil anomaly
C. Duane's retraction syndrome
D. Mobius syndrome

22. **Duane's syndrome is more common on :**
A. Left eye B. Right eye
C. Both eyes equal D. Unpredictable

23. **Brown syndrome simulates paralysis of :**
A. Sup.oblique B. Inf.oblique
C. Inferior rectus D. Superior rectus

24. **A 3-year old girl presents with fever, eyepain, periorbital swelling, proptosis and rhinorrhoea. The most likely diagnosis is :**
A. Acute frontal sinusitis
B. Acute ethmoiditis
C. Viral orbital cellulitis
D. Retinoblastoma

25. **Which of the following pigmentations of the cornea is associated least with pathologic conditions of eye or body :**
A. Fleischer ring B. Kruckenberg spindle
C. Ferry line D. Kruckenberg spindle

26. **On schiotz tonometry, it is customary to start with ——— gm weight :**
A. 3.5 B. 5.5
C. 7.5 D. 10

27. **Myriads of tiny, fine, punctate vacuoles present withing the corneal epithelium is characteristic of :**
A. Fleck dystrophy
B. Meesmann's dystrophy
C. Schnyder's crystalline dystrophy
D. Cornea farinata

28. **A 5-cm object is located 25 cm to the left of a +3.00 sph lens. The linear magnification is :**
A. 2 B. 3
C. 4 D. 5

29. **Painless, superior, palpebral corneal thinning marked by lipid deposition at the advancing edge and superficial vascularization is most characteristic of :**
A. Maren's ulcer
B. Furrow degeneration
C. Terrien's degeneration
D. Pellucid marginal degeneration

30. **The usual age at which myopia first becomes apparent is ——— years :**
A. 3 B. 8
C. 15 D. 20

31. **Pseudodendrites are associated with :**
A. Adenoviral keratitis B. Amyloidosis of cornea
C. Cystinosis of cornea D. Soft contact lens wear

32. **Cayenne Pepper spots are seen in ——— :**
A. Marfan's syndrome B. Schamberg's disease
C. Down's syndrome D. Niemann Pick's disease

33. **Syphilitic retinitis is also called ——— retinitis :**
A. Coat's B. Jacobson's
C. Jensen's D. Disciform

34. **Tay's spots on retina are ——— coloured :**
A. Pink B. Cherry red
C. White D. Golden

35. **The overall cell ratio in bipolar cones is :**
A. 1 : 2 B. 1 : 5
C. 5 : 1 D. 2 :3

36. **Extravasation of blood within the retina is ——— retinitis :**
A. Gravidic B. Leukemic
C. Apoplectic D. Renal

37. **Bipolar rods ratio is ——— :**
A. 1 : 25 B. 1 : 50
C. 1 : 125 D. 1 : 250

38. **Cotton wool spots may be seen in :**
A. Hypothyroidism B. Grave's disease
C. SLE D. None of the above

39. **Roth's spots on retina are oval——— coloured :**
A. White B. Red
C. Blue D. Yellow

40. **Blind spot is also known as ——— spot :**
A. Roth's B. Soemmering's
C. Mariotte D. Tay's

41. **Jensen's retinitis is :**
A. Renal retinopathy
B. Leukemic retinopathy
C. Diabetic retinopathy
D. Retino choroiditis juxtapapillaris

42. **A patient with manifest strabismus has his deviation neutralized with a 20-PD base-out prism OS coupled with a 10-PD base-up prism OD in primary gaze. The diagnosis is :**
A. Esotropia 20 PD with right hypertropia 1 OPHD
B. Esotropia 20 PD with left hypertropia 10 PD
C. Exotropia 20 PD with left hypertropia 10 PD
D. Exotropia 20 PD with right hypertropia 10 PD

Ans. 20. C 21. D 22. A 23. A 24. B 25. D 26. B 27. B 28. C 29. C
30. B 31. D 32. B 33. B 34. B 35. B 36. C 37. C 38. C 39. A
40. C 41. D 42. B

43. Orbital emphysema is most commonly seen with fractures of :

A. Roof of orbit
B. Floor of orbit
C. Medial wall of orbit
D. Fronta zygomatic suture

44. A lid lag on the plotic side on down gaze is characteristic of——— ptosis :

A. Traumatic B. Congenital
C. Synkinetic D. Myogenic

45. Gravidic retinitis is seen in :

A. Athletes B. Climbers
C. Divers D. Pregnancy

46. In blink response, R2 wave occurs on :

A. Same side B. Opposite side
C. Both sides D. None of the above

47. The normal accomodation of the eye which is being continuously exerted without conscious effort is —— refraction :

A. Double B. Dynamic
C. Ocular D. Static

48. Orbicularis pupillary reflex is ——— reflex :

A. Weiss's B. Westphal-Piltz
C. Preyer D. Remark's

49. Acceleration of the pulse following strong convergence of the eyeballs toward something very close to the eyes indicating sympathetic excitability is —— reflex :

A. Piltz B. Philippson's
C. Ruggeri's D. Saenger's

50. A curved reflection seen with the ophthalmoscope on the fundus of the eye to the nasal side of the disk; believed to be indicative of myopia is ——— reflex :

A. Weiss's B. Oppenheim's
C. Pusepp's D. Roger's

51. Supraorbital reflex is ——— reflex :

A. Kocher's B. Kisch's
C. McCarthy's D. McCormac's

52. Following lenticular changes occur in accomodation except :

A. Anterior pole moves forward
B. Physiological lenticonus
C. Increase in tension of lens capsule
D. Lens always moves inferiorly

53. Accomodation is well developed by the age of —— months :

A. 2 B. 6
C. 9 D. 12

54. Turnover time of water in vitreous is ——— min :

A. 5-10 B. 10-15
C. 15-20 D. 25-30

55. Predominant collagen in vitreous is type :

A. I B. II
C. III D. IC

56. Arden ratio (between the light peak and dark trough) in EOG in normal persons is usually greater than at least ———% :

A. 80 B. 120
C. 180 D. 240

57. In striate cortex, ——— layers is the thickest :

A. I B. II
C. IV D. VI

58. Vitreous weighs about ——— g:

A. 2.6 B. 3.9
C. 4.6 D. 8.2

59. Accomodative power of a 2 year old is approx. ——— diopters :

A. 15 B. 20
C. D. 28

60. 'Critical period' for acquity in humans begins at approximately ——— months :

A. 2 B. 4
C. 6 D. 8

61. Cotton-Wool spot mainly results due to :

A. Haemorrhage B. Infarction
C. Exudate D. Degeneration

62. Collier's sign is seen in :

A. Thyrotoxicosis B. Subdural haematoma
C. Midbrain disease D. Trauma

63. Which of the following is incorrectly matched about composition of human vitreous :

A. Urea—14.2 meq/100 ml
B. Lactic acid - 70 meq/100ml
C. Proteins —40 meq/L
D. Pyruvic acid —10.3 meq/L

64. The resonances in brain which cause apparent increase in brightness is knows as ——— effect :

A. Adie B. Glick
C. Broca-Sulza D. Hutchison's

65. Flickering sensation to be cone driven must be more than ——— Hz :

A. 20 B. 30
C. 40 D. 60

Ans. 43. C 44. B 45. D 46. C 47. B 48. B 49. C 50. A 51. C 52. C 53. A
54. B 55. B 56. C 57. C 58. B 59. B 60. B 61. B 62. C
63. D 64. C 65. B

66. Gene for short (blue) wavelength is found in chromosome———:
A. 7 B. 13
C. 21 D. X

67. Visual threshold increases as the subject moves from absolute darkness to very bright sunlight by a factor of ———log unit :
A. 8 B. 10
C. 12 D. 14

68. Number of classes of colour defectives is :
A. 4 B. 6
C. 8 D. 10

69. Stereopsis is poor beyond ——— from fovea :
A. 10° B. 20°
C. 30° D. 40°

70. Retina contains approx —— million rodes :
A. 30 B. 60
C. 120 D. 160

71. Optimal temporal frequency for perceiving flicker is ————Hz :
A. 8 B. 10
C. 16 D. 24

72. Vitreous does not transmit light below ——— nm :
A. 260 B. 300
C. 320 D. 360

73. Accomodationis absent by age of at least ——— years :
A. 50 B. 60
C. 65 D. 75

74. Pupillary dilatation in dark adaptation can account for an increase of sensitivity of —— log unit :
A. 0.5 B. 0.7
C. 1.3 D. 2.5

75. Lockwood's ligament connects :
A. Inferior oblique and superior oblique
B. Inferior oblique and inferior rectus
C. Superior oblique and lateral rectus
D. Superior oblique and superior rectus

76. Glands of Manz are found in :
A. Lacrimal gland B. Conjunctiva
C. Conjunctiva D. Iris

77. Most common cause of iridoplegia is :
A. Glaucoma B. Trauma
C. Keratitis D. Marfan's syndrome

78. Stocker's lines are due to :
A. Melanin B. Iron
C. Cholesterol D. Dust

79. Siegrist's spots are seen in :
A. Trachoma B. Agyrosis
C. Choroiditis D. Wilson's disease

80. Sursumversion is :
A. Elevation of one eye
B. Elevation of both eyes
C. Depression of both eyes
D. Elevation of one and depression of other eye

81. Light rays striking the retina perpendicularly are more effective in stimulating vision than those striking obliquely. This is :
A. Stiles-Granford effect B. Broca-Sulza
C. Adie's phenomenon D. Hutchison's effect

82. Titmus test is done for :
A. Corneal ulcer
B. Stereoacquity
C. Trachoma
D. Angle closure glaucoma

83. Terrien's corneal degeneration is characterized by following except :
A. Rapidly progressive
B. Young males
C. Astigmatism, against
D. Ocular perforation with minimum trauma

84. Aqueous flare is an example of ——— effect :
A. Broca Sul B. Tyndall
C. Stiles Cranford D. Hutchison's

85. Viers rod is used for :
A. Corneal foreign body
B. Angle closure glaucoma
C. Canliicular lacerations
D. Lens dislocation

86. Uhthoff's sign is seen in :
A. Diseminated sclerosis B. HIV
C. Trachoma D. Head injury

87. Circle of Zinn-Haller in formed by anastomosis of branches of ——ciliary arteries :
A. Short anterior B. Short posterior
C. Long anterior D. Long posterior

88. Jones test is used for evaluating ——— function :
A. Choroid B. Iris
C. Lacrimal D. Retinal

89. The inferior rectus is hooked in attempt to recess it 5 mm. How far from limbus will its new insertion onto sclera be —— mm :
A. 10.5 B. 11.0
C. 11.5 D. 12.7

Ans. 66. A 67. C 68. C 69. B 70. C 71. B 72. B 73. B 74. C 75. B
76. B 77. B 78. B 79. C 80. B 81. A 82. B 83. A 84. B 85. C
86. A 87. B 88. C 89. B

90. Average diurnal variation in IOP in glaucomatous eye is approx ——— mm :

A. 4 B. 6
C. 8 D. 10

91. Maximum density of rods in perifoveal region is ———mm²:

A. 30,000 B. 1,20,000
C. 1,60,000 D. 1,90,000

92. Ratio of Photoreceptors with ganglion cells is :

A. 10:1 B. 60 :1
C. 100 :1 D. 120 : 1

93. Ora Serratá is fully developed at ——— months gestational age :

A. 3 B. 6
C. 9 D. 12

94. Ciliary processes are formed at ——— months :

A. 2 B. 3
C. 6 D. 12

95. Optic vesicle is usually formed by day ——— of gestation :

A. 15 B. 25
C. 45 D. 60

96. Upper tarsal plate, centrally, is ——— times thick than that of lower one :

A. 1.0 B. 1.5
C. 2 D. 3

97. Levator muscle in an adult can raise the lid by approx ——— mm :

A. 5 B. 10
C. 15 D. 25

98. Salzman's nodular degeneration in cornea occurs following :

A. Trauma B. Trachoma
C. Glaucoma D. Marfan's syndrome

99. Krunkenberg's spindle is due to :

A. Agyrosis B. Pterygia
C. Keratoconus D. Melanin

100. Mucula retina is also called -------- spot :

A. Maxwell B. Soemmering's
C. Trousseau's D. Christopher's

101. In infancy, the eye is capable of greater than ——— D of accomodation :

A. 1 B. 14
C. 17 D. 25

102. In an emmetropic eye, the magnification is X ——— in the direct ophthalmosope :

A. 5 B. 10
C. 15 D. 25

103. The refractive powers of the following are more than that of cornea except;

A. Aquous humour
B. Crown glass
C. Crystalline lens cortex
D. Crystalline lens nucleus.

104. In contact lens correction of myopia, accomodation is needed——— than with spectacles :

A. More B. Less
C. Same D. Any of the above

105. In correction of astigmatism of more than 1 D, which of the following contact lenses are useful :

A. HEMA B. PMMA
C. Both a+b D. None

106. Wavelength of Argon Blue laser is ——— nm:

A. 418 B. 488
C. 514 D. 720

107. In essential blepharospasm, good response to botulinum, Toxin A persists for :

A. 1-2 weeks B. 2-4 weeks
C. 4-6 weeks D. 12-16 weeks

108. True about Duane's retraction syndrome is all except:

A. Unilateral
B. Diplopia common
C. Bilateral single vision is maintained by abnormal head posture
D. Esotropia

109. Duane's retraction syndrome is most common on :

A. Unilateral, Left
B. Unilateral, right
C. Bilateral but on right mor
D. Any of the above

110. In Brown's syndrome :

A. Hess chart shows no abnormally in lower field
B. Inferior oblique palsy is simulated
C. Surgery is often indicated
D. Sponataneous improvement

111. True about Tolosa-Hunt syndrome is all except :

A. Pain
B. Proptosis
C. Normal eye movement
D. Is diagnosed by CT scan

112. Collier's sign (Lid retraction) is seen in :

A. Thyrotoxicosis
B. Dorsal midbrain syndrome
C. Demyelination
D. Horner's syndrome

Ans.									
90. D	91. C	92. C	93. B	94. B	95. B	96. C	97. C	98. B	99. D
100. A,B	101. B	102. C	103. A	104. A	105. B	106. B	107. C	108. B	109. A
110. C	111. C	112.B							

113. **In nanophtalomos, the following are true except :**
A. Corneal diameter is reduced
B. Marked hypermetropia
C. Secondary angle closure glaucoma
D. Sclera is abnormally thin

114. **Reiger's syndrome has the following features except:**
A. Autosomal dominant
B. Posterior embryotoxon
C. Iris stromal hypoplasia
D. Lens opacity

115. **A patient is present which a anterior uveties, a rthritis and erythema nodosum the following are possible diagnosis except :**
A. Leprosy B. Bechcet's syndrome
C. Reiter's disease D. Crohn's disease

116. **In Ocular histoplasmosis syndrome, multifocal atrophic lesions (" Histo spots") are seen over :**
A. Sclera B. Choroid
C. Retina D. Cornea

117. **Choroidal melanoma most often spreads to:**
A. Lung B. Liver
C. Brain D. Heart

118. **Photoopthalmia is due to effect of U-V rays especially from ——— μ :**
A. 330-320 B. 311-290
C. 280-260 D. 245-230

119. **"Shortterm escape" and "long term drift" are phenomenon seen with :**
A. Pilocarpine B. Timolol
C. Physostigmine D. Atropine

120. **Ca nasopharynx most commonly involves ——— cranial nerves :**
A. III, I B. II, IV
C. IV, VI D. V, VI

121. **Paratrachoma or non-blinding trachoma is associated with —— type oculogenital chlamydial disease :**
A. A, B. C,D
C. D-K D. L-T

122. **Only upto ——— % aniseikonia is well tolerated :**
A. 1 B. 5
C. 10 D. None

123. **Astigmatism in which horizontal meridion is less curved than vertical is ——— astigmatism :**
A. With the rule B. Against the rule
C. Oblique D. Bioblique

124. **In aphakia, posterior focal point is usually ——mm behind cornea :**
A. 7 B. 14
C. 23. D. 31

125. **In aphakia, ---------- total power of eye is reduced :**
A. +6 B. +8
C. +16 D. +26

126. **On electroretinography, wave generated by Muller cells is :**
A. a B. b
C. c D. All of the above

127. **On fluorescein angiography, dye reaches the choroidal circulation —— retinal circulation :**
A. 1 second earlier B. 1 second later
C. 2 seconds earlier D. 3 seconds later

128. **Pachymeter is useful to :**
A. Study corneal endothelium
B. Study thickness of cornea
C. Measure depth of anterior chamber
D. Measure field of vision

129. **Which color would be best for foveal color testing :**
A. Red and Green B. Blue and Green
C. Yellow and Green D. Red and Blue

130. **A typical mycotic ulcer is characterized by :**
A. Elevated rolled out margins, greyish white in colour
B. Corneal vascularization
C. Big hypopyon
D. Delicate feathery finger like extensions into surrounding stroma under intact epithelium

131. **Lamellar dot sign is seen in :**
A. Congenital glaucoma B. POAG
C. Retinitis pigmentosa D. Immature cataract

122. **Following syndromes are associated with retinitis pigmentosa except :**
A. Cochayne's B. Refsum's
C. Hallgren's D. Simmond's

133. **Rhegmatogenous or primary retinal detachment is seen in ——— years and respectively :**
A. 20-40, males B. 40-60, males
C. 40-60 females D. Below 20, females

134. **Fleurettes formation is seen in :**
A. Spring catarrh B. Herpes keratitis
C. Diabetic retinopathy D. Retinoblastoma

135. **Bayneting sign is seen in :**
A. Diabetic retinopathy
B. Ciliary block glaucoma
C. POAG
D. Retinoblastoma

136. **Following drugs are commonly used for chemotherapy of retinoblastoma except :**
A. 5-FU B. Adriamycin
C. Cyclophosphamid D. Vincristine

Ans.									
113. D	114. D	115. C	116. B	117. B	118. B	119. B	120. D	121. C	122. B
123. B	124. D	125. C	126. B	127. A	128. B	129. A	130..B	131. B	132. D
133. B	134. D	135. C	136. A						

137. Visuopsychic parastriate area is :
A. 17 B. 18
C. 19 D. 20

138. Rhabdomyosarcoma of orbit most commonly arises in ——— quadrant :
A. Superior nasal B. Inferior nasal
C. Superior temporal D. Inferior temporal

139. Secondary orbital tumor is most common due to :
A. Retinoblastoma
B. Meningioma
C. Ca nasopharynx
D. Basal cell carcinoma

140. Suppurative reaction in eye is produced by following foreign body :
A. Platinum B. Nickel
C. Aluminium D. Gold

141. Optic nerve is about ——— mm in length :
A. 33-37 B. 40-43
C. 47-50 D. 55-60

142. Optic chiasma measures ——— mm horizontally :
A. 6 B. 8
C. 10 D. 12

143. In Wernicke's hemianopic pupil, ——— light reflex is absent when light is thrown on temporal half of retina of affected side and nasal half of opposite :
A. Ipsilateral direct and contralateral consensual
B. Ipsilateral direct and consensual
C. Contralateral direct and consensual
D. Contralateral direct and ipsilateral consensual

144. In ethambitol amblyopia, most common visual defect is :
A. Bi nasal hemianopia
B. Bitemporal hemianopia
C. Homonymous hemianopia
D. Quadrantic hemianopia

145. Following is true about congenital jerk nystagmus except :
A. Bilateral
B. Horizontal jerk
C. Rapid phase towards nasal side
D. Absent during sleep

146. Spasmus nutans usually resolves by the age of ——— years :
A. 2 B. 3
C. 6 D. 12

147. On exophthalmometry, a difference of more than ——— mm between the two eyes is considered significant :
A. 1 B. 2
C. 3 D. 4

148. When corneal involvement is there in Graves ophthalmopathy it is classed as ——— under American Thyroid Association (ATA) classification :
A. 2 B. 3
C. 4 D. 5

149. Oedema in mastoid region is seen in :
A. Panophthalmilis
B. Orbital cellulitis
C. Cavernous sinus thrombosis
D. Retinoblastoma

150. Incidence of primary open angle glaucoma (POAG) is about 1 in ——— population :
A. 100 B. 200
C. 1000 D. 4000

Ans. **137. C** **138. A** **139. C** **140. B** **141. C** **142. D** **143. A** **144. B** **145. C** **146. B** **147. B** **148. D** **149. C** **150. B**

OPHTHALMOLOGY

References Quoted

S.N.	Books
1.	Parson's **Diseases of the Eye.** Butterworth— Heinemann, Oxford.
2.	Khurana's **Ophthalmology.** New Age Publisher (P) Ltd., Delhi
3.	Chatterjee's **Handbook of Ophthalmology.** CBS Publishers & Distributors Pvt. Ltd., Delhi..
4.	Bhatia's **Quick Medical Text Review.** CBS Publishers & Distributors Pvt. Ltd., Delhi.

Unforgetable Supplement

Bhatia's **Quick Medical Text Review Series** (Quick revision of all the subjects in short time. No need to underline the books (read important points). CBS Publishers & Distributors Pvt. Ltd., Delhi.